Health Care in Asia

A Comparative Study of Cost and Financing

WORLD BANK REGIONAL AND SECTORAL STUDIES

Health Care in Asia

A Comparative Study of Cost and Financing

CHARLES C. GRIFFIN

The World Bank
Washington, D.C.

First printing April 1992

The World Bank Regional and Sectoral Studies series provides an outlet for work that is relatively limited in its subject matter or geographical coverage but that contributes to the intellectual foundations of development operations and policy formulation. These studies have not necessarily been edited with the same rigor as Bank publications that carry the imprint of a university press.

The findings, interpretations, and conclusions expressed in this publication are those of the authors and should not be attributed in any manner to the World Bank, to its affiliated organizations, or to the members of its Board of Executive Directors or the countries they represent.

The complete backlist of publications from the World Bank is shown in the annual *Index of Publications*, which contains an alphabetical title list and indexes of subjects, authors, and countries and regions. The latest edition is available free of charge from Distribution Unit, Office of the Publisher, The World Bank, 1818 H Street, N.W., Washington, D.C. 20433, U.S.A., or from Publications, The World Bank, 66, avenue d'Iéna, 75116 Paris, France.

Charles C. Griffin is a senior research associate with the Urban Institute while on leave from his position as associate professor of economics at the University of Oregon.

Cover design by Sam Ferro

Library of Congress Cataloging-in-Publication Data

Griffin, Charles C., 1951–
Health care in Asia : a comparative study of cost and financing /
Charles C. Griffin
p. cm.—(World Bank regional and sectoral studies)
Includes bibliographical references.
ISBN 0-8213-2055-6
1. Medical care, Cost of—Asia 2. Medical economics—Asia.
I. Title. II. Series.
RA410.55.A78G75 1992
338.4'33621'095—dc20 92-2216
CIP

Contents

Text tables

Appendix tables

Text figures

Appendix figures

Boxes

Foreword

This study on health in Asia by Charles Griffin and the companion study on education by Jee-Peng Tan and Alain Mingat (forthcoming) were initiated in 1988 as complements to other World Bank studies on the social sectors. As chief economist in the Asia Region at that time, I launched these studies to help strengthen the factual and analytical basis of the World Bank's lending operations in the Asia Region in two sectors that relate directly to the Bank's broader concern with poverty alleviation.

Both studies provide an overview of sectoral development, with an emphasis on cost and finance issues. This focus was chosen because education and health outcomes depend critically on resource allocation in the sectors, and allocation, in turn, is influenced by policy choices affecting costs and finance. The studies share three aims: to document current patterns of costs, finance, and outcomes in individual Asian countries; to explore linkages between sectoral performance and policy choices; and to identify potential policy options to promote efficient and equitable sectoral development.

The studies rest on a rich data base compiled from varied sources. While some of the data can be found in widely available publications (such as United Nations Yearbooks), other data, particularly on cost and finance, are scarcer. For the latter, the authors have drawn on documents provided by governments in the context of the Bank's operational activity. In this task, the contribution of colleagues in the Asia Region has been critical, for their generosity in sharing materials acquired in the course of their own work made it possible for the authors to assemble as much data as they have. Beyond this, the studies have also benefited from extensive discussion among Asia Region staff, so that they are, in a sense, a product of collaborative effort among Bank staff to expand knowledge and understanding of education and health issues in the region.

Comparative analysis was the common approach in both studies, with countries rather than individuals as the unit of observation. This orientation allows the authors to examine the impact of system-wide policies—such as the extent of private financing in a system—on sectoral development. Asian countries, and probably countries in other regions as well, differ widely in policy choices as well as in outcomes. The diversity permits assessment of individual countries' performance relative to others in the region and sheds light on the possible range of alternative policy choices and options. It also invites exploration of the linkages between policies and outcomes.

Several basic themes emerge repeatedly in the study on health. Asia's overall progress in improving health and reducing fertility has compared favorably with that of other regions of the world. But within Asia there is tremendous variability in performance. In the poorly performing countries, health problems continue to be connected to the same infectious and parasitic diseases that have dominated health problems in Asia for centuries. These countries have fast-growing populations, so expanding cohorts of children and of women of childbearing age will continue to bear the burden of unhealthy living conditions. Emphasis on health programs that give children a healthy start in life and ensure that they can live in environments relatively free from preventable diseases should be a major concern. In addition, the persistent excess mortality for women in South Asia is a serious problem that merits considerable attention by government. Countries that have enjoyed fast-improving health indicators over the last two decades are already reorienting their financing to the needs of older and healthier populations, but infectious and parasitic diseases continue to pose serious threats to some groups.

There is considerable variability in how the health sector is financed as well. First, a handful of countries (accounting, however, for nearly 400 million people) have lagged considerably behind their neighbors in improving infant mortality and life expectancy at birth. These countries, including Bangladesh, Indonesia, Nepal, and the Philippines, have also lagged in public spending in the health sector and have poorly allocated what they spend.

Second, most countries in the sample have tapped a narrow financial base for financing government health services. Of the three possible sources of revenue—taxes, insurance, and private out-of-pocket spending—most government systems are almost completely dependent on taxes. Many of them could broaden the health sector's base by introducing user fees and some form of health insurance. A greater role for the private sector would be facilitated in many countries by such changes.

Third, governments usually argue that fairness and redistributive considerations are important elements of public spending for health care. Thus one would expect to find that relatively more public resources would be devoted to poorer areas and to areas with higher infant mortality rates. It appears from this study that most do not. Much better targeting of public sector spending is certainly feasible for the countries included in this study.

A theme that emerges from the findings, with regard to both health conditions and financing, is that the health sector would benefit if governments paid more attention to public or community health activities whose benefits extend beyond the individual. Doing so may mean spending more tax money in some countries. It probably means reallocating public spending in all countries, and this reallocation would be facilitated by turning over some tax-financed activities to the private sector or to other forms of finance. However, shifting the emphasis in spending from curative health care to public health programs is a political economy issue. Those who benefit most from curative services—hospital administrators, physicians, nurses, and adults whose interest is motivated by acute illness—are likely to continue to dominate the competition for scarce resources. The benefits to any single individual from public health care are small, so advocacy for public health spending tends to be voluntary, poorly organized, and intermittent. The author urges donors to counterbalance spending patterns created by these internal pressures on developing country governments, especially in South Asia. A greater emphasis on community health activities by government is likely to improve economic efficiency, equity, and health—an attractive set of outcomes for any policy reform.

Beyond these broad messages, the reader will find ample information about Asian health in this study, as well as analytical support for the foregoing conclusions. It is my hope that the study's publication in an easily accessible form will contribute to a lively discussion among policymakers and others regarding future directions for development of the health sector in Asian countries, thereby encouraging consideration of policies to build on Asia's remarkable progress in the sector.

Oktay Yenal
Chief, India Resident Mission
Asia Region

Acknowledgments

I am delighted to acknowledge other contributors to this project. Many people in the Asia Region at the World Bank assisted in this enterprise by carefully assembling statistics for the countries examined here, and many discussed with me what they hoped an investigation such as this one would accomplish. This study would not have been possible without their contributions of ideas, background documents, and reviews. Andrea Madarassy worked for about seven months as a research assistant on this project. She assembled most of the data and created an entirely new data base on insurance. I greatly appreciate her inputs and insights. Jose Martins, Susan Stout, and Oktay Yenal read several versions and provided constructive comments that led to improvements in both the content and the presentation. I also received helpful comments on an earlier version from Willy de Geyndt, Joseph Kutzin, Maureen Lewis, Vic Paqueo, Alexander ter Weele, and Julia Walsh. Four anonymous reviewers provided additional detailed critiques to which I have responded in this final version. To all of these colleagues, my warm regards and thanks. I have tried to use their ideas to improve the manuscript, but I will let them decide whether I succeeded.

My greatest debt is to Jee-Peng Tan, who developed this project and offered me this piece to write. She and Alain Mingat have written a companion piece on education in Asia (forthcoming). I have benefited from her talent for breaking complex tasks into manageable components and from her ability to tease meaningful themes from available numbers. Her detective's instinct for tracking down statistics and publications has contributed materially to the quality of this paper. She read several drafts of it carefully and rewrote some sections. I appreciate the opportunity to have worked with her.

Editorial and production support was provided by Alison Strong (editing), Kim Bieler (desktopping), and Kathy Rosen (graphics).

1

Introduction

If the 1970s are remembered as a decade in which ambitious goals for providing basic health services and reducing population growth rates were widely promulgated, the 1980s will be remembered for the stark realization that those activities are expensive and among the first to be cut when economic growth falters. In Asia, where economic performance has been unusually strong during the past decade and even the poorest economies have shown striking resilience, governments have not escaped difficult decisions about resource allocation in the social sectors. In the poorer Asian countries, persistent burdens of poverty, poor health, and high population growth have strained resources in the health sector. In wealthier countries that have made great improvements in health and fertility outcomes, the resulting change in age structure and morbidity patterns portends even greater financial demands on the health sector.

Asia's achievements in health and fertility over the last two decades have been impressive. This book addresses the question of how improved financing of those sectors could help governments to build on that performance. Even the poorest countries have shared in this trend—although at a somewhat slower pace than their neighbors. In India, for example, which had a per capita income of about US$300 in 1986, life expectancy at birth has increased nearly 30 percent in two decades, to 57 years. Its life expectancy exceeds that reached 45 years ago in Japan, whose per capita income then was considerably higher than that in India today. China, Indonesia, the Republic of Korea, and Thailand have experienced significant reductions in fertility rates during the last 20 years. Their performance signals a transition to lower population growth rates, better health for mothers and children, and greater human capital investments in the young.

This report assembles data on health, demographic trends, health infrastructure, health personnel, and health financing across Asian countries. In a broad and imprecise manner, it attempts to relate differences in spending priorities and patterns to health outcomes. This effort should be viewed as a complement to country-specific and household-level analysis. Although some interesting patterns and trends—as well as one or two surprising empirical regularities—arise in the data, at the level of aggregation used in this report it is virtually impossible to attribute causation to the relations that unfold.

Although it is easy to criticize an effort such as this one—because of such problems as the questionable comparability of numbers across countries, the imprecision of many of the statistics, the unobservable intervening activities that take place between a budget allocation and the delivery of services, and the different physical environments within which health policies operate—cross-national comparisons are valuable for understanding the general direction of health policy.

Two examples of the value of this aggregative approach can be given. First, large differences in health outcomes across Asian countries are documented in this report. Asian countries that started at a low level of health in 1965 tended to be in an even worse position relative to their neighbors by the 1980s. Nevertheless, there are success stories that could provide guidance for changing this trend in the 1990s. Second, large differences across Asian countries in the mix of public and private spending are reported. Countries at either end of that distribution might consider policies that would change the mix. Countries with a high proportion of private spending might benefit from higher spending on public health activities that are not efficiently provided through private markets. Countries with high public spending are probably displacing some private spending. In each of these examples, *high* and *low* are relative terms. We have no knowledge of the correct level of spending, the correct mix of spending from different sources, or the highest achievable level of health for a given GNP, but we can get an idea of reasonable values for these ranges by comparing countries.

Cautionary notes

Some categories or labels used in this paper may be questioned by experts in specific countries. One particularly problematic term is insurance. Is insurance in Korea the same as insurance in China? Probably not. In Korea insurance is compulsory for much of the population but is administered through insurance funds. In China employers must provide insurance to their employees, but there is little risk-sharing among employers. Yet there are also private insurance funds and village-level insurance plans that are clearly risk-sharing arrangements. In other countries, such as Malaysia and Papua New Guinea, formal insurance is provided only by the private sector. Although health insurance is poorly developed, it is based on voluntary arrangements for employee groups through private underwriters. Yet those two countries in effect provide health insurance to the vast majority of their populations through the provision of medical services in the government sector, which, although never called insurance, has the same impact.

There are other problems, such as whether spending on military health care is included in central government health spending and to what degree spending by lower levels of government is included, if at all. For a study of this kind, we are dependent on the definitions used by those who put the original data together. Almost by default, if they call something insurance, that is what it is called here. Military spending is rarely, if ever, reported as part of government health spending, so it will usually not be included in figures presented in this paper. Central and local government expenditure on health has been estimated for many countries, but it would be misleading to say that the numbers presented in this report are comprehensive. However, none of the conclusions drawn from the evidence is so strong as to be dependent on whether these problems of nomenclature or data are completely resolved.

How accurate are the numbers? They are the best available in 1989. Some are the best available in 1990. The farther back we go, the less reliable the estimates become. The accuracy of financial and health statistics has improved markedly since the mid-1970s, and the World Bank's increasing interest in the social sectors is a key reason for the improvement. There are many problems even with such commonly used statistics as those on life expectancy and infant mortality, but the improvement in their comparability and accuracy has been enormous in the last 20 years.

Organization of the study

Chapter 2 reviews mortality data, medical inputs, and health expenditure for regions of the world for the mid-1980s. When statistics are available for both 1965 and 1986, trends are examined as well. The same variables are reviewed for the Asian countries included in this study. Chapter 3 attempts to construct a health profile for the developing countries of Asia using cause-of-death information, the age structure of the populations, and related evidence. Chapter 4 reviews the data that could be assembled for 1986 or 1987 on sources of health expenditure, health infrastructure, and related financial data for countries in the sample. Chapter 5 discusses user fees and insurance, the two main alternatives to tax financing of public sector curative services. Chapter 6 pieces together information from many sources in an attempt to assess the degree to which public subsidies in the health sector are targeted, and to whom. Chapter 7 reviews the main themes.

This is an inductive, exploratory study. It is demanding of the reader in that the available evidence is presented in detail. The evidence has been put within a structure designed to help make sense of it, and tentative conclusions are drawn in terms of that structure, but readers are given the ammunition to make their own judgments. Readers expecting firm conclusions based on rigorous analysis of good data will be disappointed. The objective of the study is to assemble data essential for making sensible public policy decisions in the health sector, data that should be readily available but rarely are. Building on the evidence assembled in this volume should be the highest priority, both within countries and across countries. Readers are challenged to take points of disagreement and holes in the evidence as opportunities to push this study to the next step.

2

Current Health Conditions

World comparisons

In contrast to education, in which progress can be measured almost yearly by enrollment ratios, performance on standardized tests, completion rates, and rates of return, measuring progress in health and population is less clear-cut. Life expectancy and fertility rates, for example, are slow to change. And changes result from a variety of causes, including increases in income, knowledge, and government and private activities. The roles played by specific health interventions are difficult to pinpoint.

Because of the difficulty of isolating the effects of programs on such outcomes, health and family planning programs are often evaluated in terms of their intermediate outputs—such as immunization coverage or contraceptive use rates—and their inputs. Cross-country comparisons of the availability of inputs, such as population per physician, are used as indicators of differing conditions across countries, but the relative importance of each input to better health is subject to debate.

This chapter distinguishes among measures of health and population outcomes, the intermediate outputs or process variables (such as immunizations), physical inputs, and expenditure in comparing the performance and activity levels of different countries and regions. In addition, comparisons are made in both the current state of those variables and changes in them.

Outcomes in 1986

There are still differences in female life expectancy at birth among developing regions (table 2.1). Asia lags behind Latin America by 6 years, and Africa lags behind Asia by 10 years. All the developing regions lag behind the industrial countries, where female life expectancy is 10 to 26 years longer. Although female life expectancy at birth in Asia, Latin America, and Europe, the Middle East, and North Africa has exceeded 60 years, in 1986 it lagged behind the average level achieved by industrial nations in 1965 by 7 to 10 years. Women tend to live longer than men in all

Table 2.1 Health and fertility indicators by region, 1986

Country group	*Life expectancy at birth (years)* Female	*Life expectancy at birth (years)* Male	*Infant mortality rate (per 1,000)*	*Child mortality rate (per 1,000)*	*Total fertility rate (children per woman)*	*Woman's lifetime chance of death in childbirth (percent)*
Asia	63	62	60	63	4.4	1.41
Africa	53	49	110	83	6.5	7.06
Europe, Middle East, and North Africa	63	60	76	144	6.2	4.97
Latin America	69	63	56	23	3.7	0.65
Industrial countries	79	73	9	0.53	1.8	0.02

Note: Data are weighted by population.
Source: Appendix tables A.2 and A.3.

regions, but the differences vary from only 1 year in Asia to 6 years in Latin America and the industrial countries.

Much of the difference in life expectancy is embedded in differences in infant and child mortality rates (table 2.1).[1] Among developing regions, Asia has done well in both infant and child mortality. Its infant mortality rate exceeds Latin America's rate by only 7 percent, but its child mortality rate is much higher. These two measures are age-specific components of life expectancy that can be targeted with known, effective interventions (such as health inputs for mothers before and during birth, immunizations, oral rehydration therapy, birth spacing, and nutrition supplements).

Comparisons of the total fertility rate[2] indicate differences in performance in controlling population growth. Asian countries, with Latin America, have the lowest fertility for the developing regions of the world, but the rate is approximately double replacement fertility.[3] Large cohorts of women will enter their childbearing years in the next several decades in Asia. This will result in continued high population growth rates in the region, which already accounts for more than half the world's population.

The measure of the probability that a woman will die in childbirth in her lifetime captures the interaction of high fertility rates and poor health conditions as they affect the riskiness of childbirth (table 2.1). The probability that a woman will die in childbirth is low across the world in absolute terms, but there are huge differences among regions. Women in Asia are about 70 times more likely to die in childbirth than women in industrial countries; and women in Africa are about 5 times more likely to die in childbirth than women in Asia.

Changes in outcomes, 1965–86

The Asian countries exceeded all other regions in improving female life expectancy and infant mortality in 1965–86 (table 2.2). There are somewhat larger differences in improvements in child mortality, with Asia clearly lagging behind Africa and Latin

Table 2.2 Change in health and fertility indicators by region, 1965–86
(percent)

Country group	Life expectancy at birth (years): Female	Life expectancy at birth (years): Male	Infant mortality rate (per 1,000)	Child mortality rate (per 1,000)	Total fertility rate (children per woman)
Asia	25	29	-51	-14	-29
Africa	19	19	-30	-32	-0.9
Europe, Middle East, and North Africa	17	15	-43	-19	-11
Latin America	16	13	-42	-50	-35
Industrial countries	7	7	-62	-48	-34

Note: These figures are sensitive to the absolute size of the statistics in 1965. For example, a drop in the infant mortality rate from 20 to 15 is a 25 percent decline. A drop from 100 to 95, the same in absolute terms, is only a 5 percent decline.
Source: Appendix tables A.2 and A.3.

America. The surprisingly strong performance of the industrial countries in reducing infant mortality from the already low levels in 1965 suggests that there are opportunities for great progress in this area. The same could be said for the total fertility rate, for which the largest declines were in the industrial countries (although Asia was close behind).

Process variables, 1986

Table 2.3 contains measures of intermediate outputs (or indices of program effort) by region for the most recent year. The first column shows the percentage of one-year-olds receiving a full series of diphtheria-pertussis-tetanus (DPT) immunizations. It is a reasonably good measure of the efficacy of immunization programs because a complete three-shot DPT sequence represents a considerable motivational and logistical achievement for health systems in many countries. Similarly, increasing the percentage of births attended by a trained birth attendant is an important input for both health and population programs but requires substantial improvements in health infrastructure in rural areas as well as changes in mothers' behavior.

Although the accuracy of the numbers in table 2.3 is likely to be poor, it is nevertheless clear that the 1980s saw large improvements in immunization coverage in developing regions as new programs were started. But the large percentage changes have often been from low starting points. In Asia, for example, only 43 percent of one-year-olds received the full series of DPT shots in 1986, but that represents a 154 percent improvement in just five years. Further expanding coverage, then sustaining it for each new cohort of babies, is a difficult task that has yet to be tested in most developing countries. If these improvements are maintained, however, they should begin strongly to affect child mortality and morbidity in the near future.[4]

Inputs

Asia has high population-to-physician and population-to-nurse ratios that have improved at a rate about average for the world (table 2.4). Much of the improvement in these ratios took place in the 1980s, with the change in physician and nursing personnel in the first 5 years of the 1980s nearly matching the performance of the previous 15 years. Asian (and African) countries have substituted some lower-level personnel for physicians, which shows up clearly in the ratios between regions: relative to Latin America, Asia has 2.4 times more people per physician but 1.9 times more people per nurse. The improvements in health and population outcomes for Asia shown in the previous tables have been accomplished with relatively small supplies of physicians and nursing personnel.

Health expenditure

Asia's combined public and private medical expenditure per capita is nearly as low as Africa's (table 2.5). Even the relatively high spending in Latin America and Europe, the Middle East, and North Africa is less than 5 percent of spending in industrial countries. The large improvements in health and population outcomes that have been achieved in the developing world have cost relatively little, but the experience of the industrial countries indicates that additional improvements may require higher and higher per capita expenditure.

Spending on health care by central governments in Asia was approximately 3 percent of their budgets, which is near the low end of the scale. It translates into central government spending of about $2.3 per capita in the mid-1980s.[5] Although the figures for total and central government per capita spending in table 2.5 are not strictly comparable, the low figure for Asia suggests high private expenditure in that region on health relative to other regions. Asia and Africa both spend, in total,

Table 2.3 Intermediate outputs of health and fertility programs by region, 1986
(percent)

Country group	*One-year-olds immunized with full DPT cycle*	*Change in coverage of full DPT cycle 1981–86*	*Births attended by trained personnel*
Asia	43	154	46
Africa	37	303	47
Europe, Middle East, and North Africa	34	728	46
Latin America	58	543	63
Industrial countries	65	22	99

Note: Trained personnel refers to physicians, nurses, and midwives with formal training, but excludes traditional midwives.
Source: Appendix table A.4.

Table 2.4 Population per physician and nurse by region, 1984

Country group	Population per physician 1984	Change in population per physician (percent) 1965–84	Population per nurse 1984	Change in population per nurse (percent) 1965–84
Asia	2,894	-43	1,932	-56
Africa	22,657	-32	2,082	-54
Europe, Middle East, and North Africa	774	-49	1,651	-58
Latin America	1,215	-47	1,011	-32
Industrial countries	470	-41	143	-63

Source: Appendix table A.4.

Table 2.5 Health expenditure per capita, by region, 1986

Country group	Per capita private and government health expenditure (U.S. dollars)	Central government expenditure devoted to health (percent)	Per capita central government expenditure on health (U.S. dollars)	Health expenditure as percentage of GDP (government and private)	Countries with data
Asia	13	2.9	2.3	3.1	9
Africa	12	5.4	5.3	3.2	19
Europe, Middle East, and North Africa	51	2.1	13.4	5.7	11
Latin America	69	4.8	22.9	5.8	18
Industrial countries	1,312	11.6	447.0	11.3	20

Note: Data are calculated from national accounts estimates of medical care consumption. The numbers come from the International Comparison Project and use purchasing power parities. These figures are the best available for comparing expenditure across countries, but they have been calculated for only 79 countries and refer in most cases to a year before 1985.
Source: Appendix table A.1.

roughly $13 per capita on health care. The central government accounts for about 18 percent of that spending in Asia, but 44 percent in Africa. Central governments in Latin America and in Europe, the Middle East, and North Africa account for 44 and 27 percent of spending, respectively. Total spending on health care as a percentage of GDP is lowest in Asia, so the region's good performance in health indicators has been achieved at a relatively low cost.

Conclusion

The foregoing comparisons must be viewed conservatively. Nevertheless, they indicate that progress in improving health and reducing population growth rates has been strong in Asia over the last 20 years. Asia is not exceptional: the same could be said of Latin America and Europe, the Middle East, and North Africa. Small differences in regional averages for most outcome measures, despite large differences in spending and inputs for these three regions, suggest that there are many different methods that can achieve similar results. Africa lags behind the other regions and is the outlier for every measure.

One of the most surprising findings from these tables is the large *percentage* improvement in health outcomes in industrial countries during the last 20 years despite the high levels of good health they had already achieved by 1965. Continued improvement in health outcomes in industrial countries is consistent with the notion of decreasing returns to additional spending on health care because the improvement has been purchased at extraordinary cost. Although the standard of good health produced by industrial countries (infant mortality at or below 10 per thousand, female life expectancy at birth of about 80 years) will improve slowly because of the decreasing productivity of additional inputs, it will nevertheless continue to improve as more and more resources are devoted to health care in those countries.

Developing countries consequently face a moving target in the definition of good health. Yet, on the basis of the experiences of Europe and North America, we can expect that the decreasing returns to health spending in terms of reductions in mortality will be offset by rapidly rising medical expenditure in the newly industrializing countries of Asia. The International Comparison Project estimates that each 1 percent increase in per capita GDP across countries results in a 1.4 percent increase in per capita health expenditure. Medical expenditure will consequently grow at a much faster clip than per capita GNP in Asia.

Comparisons within Asia

Outcomes in 1986

The averages cited above mask large differences within Asia; in fact, for nearly every measure, differences within Asia are larger than those across world regions. Table 2.6 shows the performance in Asian countries in the outcome variables. Two region-wide averages are shown for each measure at the bottom of this and subsequent tables: one that does not take population into account and one that is weighted by population. In most cases the two averages are within a few points of each other; both are shown because of the heavy weight of China and India in the population-weighted numbers.

The range in female life expectancy across these countries exceeds 25 years, from 47 in Nepal to 73 in Korea. Infant mortality ranges from a low of 25 per thousand live births in Korea to a high of 130 in Nepal. There is an even larger difference in child mortality between these two countries. While Nepal's infant mortality rate is about 5 times Korea's, its child mortality rate is nearly 11 times Korea's. The total fertility rate ranges from 2.2 in Korea to 5.9 in Nepal.

Table 2.6 Health and fertility indicators in selected Asian countries, 1986

Country	Life expectancy at birth (years) F	M	F–M	Infant mortality rate (per 1,000)	Child mortality rate (per 1,000)	Total fertility rate (children per woman)	Woman's lifetime chance of death in childbirth (percent)
Bangladesh	50	51	-1	121	78	5.6	4.0
China	70	68	2	34	12	2.3	0.1
India	56	57	-1	86	55	4.4	2.6
Indonesia	58	55	3	87	46	3.6	3.4
Korea	73	66	7	25	7	2.2	0.1
Malaysia	71	67	4	27	9	3.5	0.3
Myanmar	61	58	3	64	24	4.4	0.7
Nepal	47	48	-1	130	78	5.9	5.9
Papua New Guinea	54	51	3	64	23	5.2	6.1
Philippines	65	62	3	46	29	4.6	0.4
Sri Lanka	72	68	4	29	10	2.9	0.3
Thailand	66	62	4	41	10	3.0	1.0
Country average	62	59	3	63	32	4.0	2.1
Population-weighted	63	62	1	60	33	3.4	1.4

F = female, M = male.
Source: World Bank 1988c, and Ross and others 1988.

Several pairs of countries that have similar per capita incomes, such as Indonesia and the Philippines or China and India, show divergent performances in these measures. Both China and Sri Lanka have achieved health and fertility levels that compare favorably with those in industrial countries. Male life expectancy at birth lags behind female life expectancy by about three years on average in the Asian sample, but in Bangladesh, India, and Nepal, men live longer than women on average. In China, women outlive men by about two years, but this number compares unfavorably with that in other Asian countries with similar life expectancies, where women outlive men by three to seven years.

The estimates of the percentage chance that a woman facing the average total fertility and maternal mortality rates will die in childbirth are imprecise, so small differences among countries are probably meaningless. Yet the differences between some countries with otherwise similar conditions are extraordinary (table 2.6). A woman in India faces a 2.6 percent chance of dying in childbirth compared with only a 0.1 percent chance in China. The odds of dying in childbirth are higher in Thailand than in the Philippines, despite Thailand's lower fertility rate. In a disturbingly large proportion of the countries (including a large share of the total population of Asia outside China—in Bangladesh, India, Indonesia, Nepal, and Papua New Guinea), the odds of a woman dying in childbirth during her lifetime are better than 2 in 100. Although even the highest probabilities are low in an absolute sense, nearly all the deaths are preventable, and they will be reduced as countries lower fertility and infant mortality rates. In South Asia the problem of maternal mortality is large enough to cause female mortality to exceed male mortality during the otherwise healthy middle years, giving rise to the shorter life expectancies for women that are evident in table 2.6.

Changes in outcomes, 1965–86

Several countries with low levels of life expectancy in 1965, such as Nepal and Bangladesh, experienced relatively small improvements in life expectancy between 1965 and 1986 (table 2.7). Other countries, such as the Philippines and Thailand, also improved at a slow rate but from much higher initial levels of life expectancy.[6] One result is that a fast-improving country like Papua New Guinea, which had the same female life expectancy as Bangladesh in 1965, had one four years longer in 1986. Korea and Thailand had the same female life expectancies in 1965, but by 1986 a newborn female in Korea would live seven years longer on average than her contemporary in Thailand (a 10 percent longer life). Despite low per capita GNP, China had

Table 2.7 Change in health and fertility indicators in selected Asian countries, 1965–86
(percent)

Country	*Change in female life expectancy at birth*	*Change in infant mortality rate*	*Change in child mortality rate*	*Change in total fertility rate*
Bangladesh	14	-21	-24	-18
China	25	-62	-67	-64
India	27	-43	-50	-29
Indonesia	29	-36	-51	-35
Korea	26	-60	-65	-54
Malaysia	18	-51	-63	-44
Myanmar	25	-48	-58	-24
Nepal	18	-29	-32	-2
Papua New Guinea	23	-54	-68	-16
Philippines	14	-36	-40	-32
Sri Lanka	11	-54	-63	-40
Thailand	14	-53	-74	-52
Country average	20	-46	-54	-34
Population-weighted	25	-51	-57	-46

Source: World Bank 1988c, and Ross and others 1988.

extraordinary success over the period in improving life expectancy; it was more than 70 years by 1986. China's success is clearly related to large improvements in infant and child mortality.

The other health indicators are consistent with the overall trend in life expectancy. Most of the group are within 10 points of the average reduction in both infant mortality and child mortality. The countries that had already achieved relatively low infant and child mortality by 1965 continued to experience large percentage improvements in those indicators, far greater than the increase in life expectancy in these countries. However, several middle-income countries whose progress was slower than the group average, particularly Indonesia and the Philippines, fell behind other countries that had higher infant mortality rates in 1965. In 1965, for example, the Philippines' infant mortality rate was 88 percent of Thailand's; by 1986, it was 112 percent of Thailand's.

Total fertility rates fell sharply over the period. China, Korea, and Thailand led the way, with reductions of more than 50 percent in two decades. Only Nepal failed to achieve a double-digit decline.

Changes in process variables

DPT immunization coverage in 1986 exceeded 50 percent in all countries except Bangladesh, Myanmar, Nepal, and Papua New Guinea (table 2.8). Improvements in immunization coverage for one-year-olds during the 1980s were substantial for most of the countries in the sample, but the large percentage increases for the countries with low coverage rates resulted because immunization programs in these countries have only recently gotten under way. Bangladesh, for example, increased coverage by 800 percent, but immunized only 9 percent of infants in 1986.

Countries that experienced significant declines in fertility also attained high contraceptive prevalence rates,[7] but there is not a one-to-one correspondence between the two variables. For example, Myanmar and Papua New Guinea realized lower fertility rates and larger declines in fertility than did Bangladesh and Nepal, despite lower contraceptive prevalence rates.

In South Asian countries other than Sri Lanka, a third or fewer of all births were attended by trained health personnel for the years around 1984.

Inputs

The ratios of physicians[8] and nurses to population improved in all the sample countries between 1965 and 1984, although improvement has been slow (and recent) in Bangladesh, Papua New Guinea, the Philippines, and Sri Lanka (table 2.9). The ratio of nurses to physicians is another concern. In industrial countries, there are roughly three nurses to one physician in curative systems requiring relatively intensive use of physician services. In Bangladesh, one of the countries in Asia with the greatest shortage of personnel, there are actually fewer nurses than physicians. The ratio of

Table 2.8 Health and fertility process variables in selected Asian countries, 1986
(percent)

Country	*One-year-olds immunized with full DPT cycle*	*Change in coverage for full DPT cycle 1981–86*	*Births attended by trained personnel*	*Modern contraceptive prevalence rate mid-1980s*
Bangladesh	9	800	..	16
China	75	..	..	77
India	58	87	33	35
Indonesia	69	..	31	42
Korea	76	25	65	52
Malaysia	59	9	82	22
Myanmar	23	360	97	5[a]
Nepal	46	188	10	14
Papua New Guinea	41	-18	34	4
Philippines	73	43	..	20
Sri Lanka	61	36	87	39
Thailand	80	54	33	66
Country average	56	158	52	33
Population-weighted	65	155	37	53

.. Not available.
a. Myanmar's entry is for all methods.
Source: Ross and others 1988, and UNICEF 1988.

nurses to physicians is also small in China and India. China's shortage is not as serious as India's because the number of physicians in China is overstated relative to other countries; in India, if anything, the number of nurses is overstated.[9] The composition of these numbers is more carefully investigated in chapter 4, but the numbers here are aggregated to be consistent with the regional statistics discussed earlier.

Differences in the ratio of nurses to physicians are definitely a matter of policy in developing countries, because governments often pay for the training of these professionals. For example, Nepal and Thailand have aggressively added physician substitutes to their health worker cadres, which has resulted in greatly improved population-to-nurse ratios in less than a decade even though there has been little or no improvement in population-to-physician ratios. Not only do governments control these numbers, but staffing levels and types of staff are also important determinants of the costs of programs and their coverage.

Relating infant mortality and female life expectancy to per capita GNP

The variation across countries in health outcomes stems partly from differences in economic circumstances, education, and other variables, but health policies are also believed to exert a significant influence. Figure 2.1 displays infant mortality rates for

Table 2.9 Population per physician and nurse in selected Asian countries, 1984

Country	*Population per physician 1984*	*Change in population per physician (percent) 1965–84*	*Population per nurse 1984*	*Change in population per nurse (percent) 1965–84*	*Ratio of nurses to physicians 1984*
Bangladesh	6,730	-17	8,980	..	0.7
China	1,000	-38	1,700	-44	0.6
India	2,520	-48	1,700	-74	1.5
Indonesia	9,460	-70	1,260	-87	5.4
Korea	1,170	-57	590	-80	2.0
Malaysia	1,930	-69	1,010	-24	2.0
Myanmar	3,740	-68	900	-92	4.2
Nepal	32,710	-29	4,680	-95	7.0
Papua New Guinea	6,160	-51	890	44	7.0
Philippines[a]	6,700	..	2,740	143	2.4
Sri Lanka	5,520	-5	1,290	-60	4.3
Thailand	6,290	-12	710	-86	8.9
Country average	6,994	-43	2,204	-41	4.0
Population-weighted	2,937	-43	1,972	-56	1.8

.. Not available.
a. Government personnel only.
Source: World Bank 1989d.

Figure 2.1 Infant mortality rate and per capita GNP, world, 1986

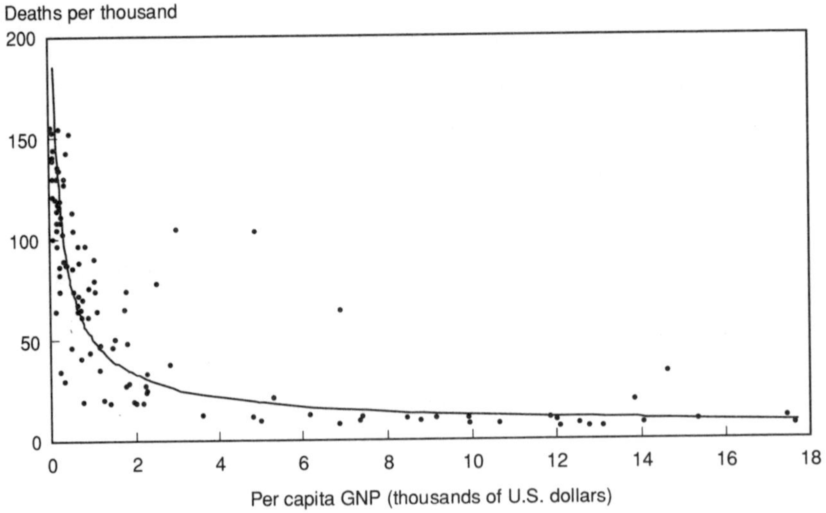

Note: The fitted line in the figure is the ordinary least-squares regression ln(IMR) = a + ln(GNP per capita).
Source: Appendix table A.2.

the world in 1986 against GNP per capita. Each dot represents one country, and a least-squares regression line is drawn through the observations. For countries with a per capita income of more than $3,000–$4,000, infant mortality presses close to the zero limit except for the few outliers. For countries with a per capita income below $3,000, however, the dispersion in performance is large, although for many a low GNP explains the infant mortality rate with great accuracy. Small *decreases* in GNP per capita at the lower end of the scale correspond to fairly large *increases* in the infant mortality rate. Figure 2.2 enlarges the lower portion of figure 2.1 and shows where the Asian countries are located. Only two countries in the sample, Papua New Guinea and Indonesia, have higher infant mortality rates than would be predicted on the basis of their GNP per capita, but there are marked differences for countries at virtually the same levels of income.

The major policy question from a cross-country perspective is: What makes the performance of China, Myanmar, and Sri Lanka so much better than other countries near the same point on the income scale? Are their experiences transferable to countries with high infant mortality? To what extent are the differences embedded in policy and financial choices that these countries have made?

In a similar fashion, figure 2.3 shows female life expectancy at birth in 1986 by level of GNP per capita. To a degree, this graph is the mirror image of the infant mortality graph, with countries with per capita GNP above $3,000–$4,000 pushing

Figure 2.2 Infant mortality rate and per capita GNP, selected Asian countries and world trend, 1986

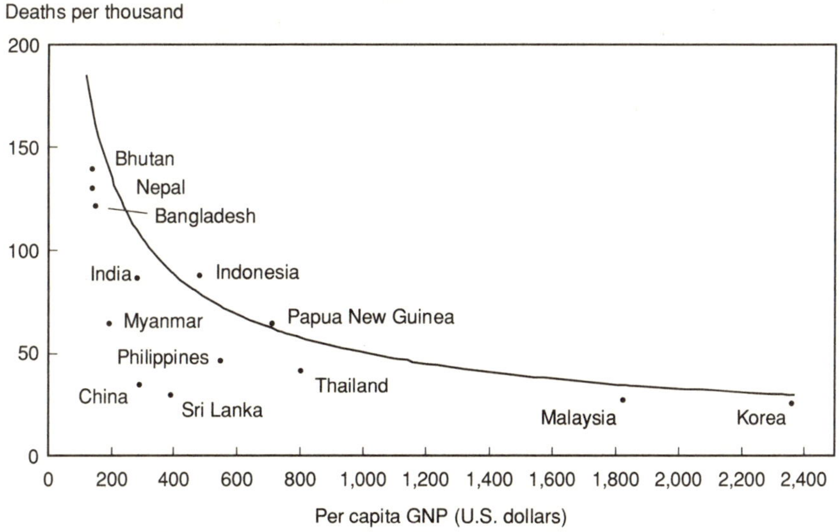

Source: Appendix table A.2.

Figure 2.3 Female life expectancy at birth and per capita GNP, world, 1986

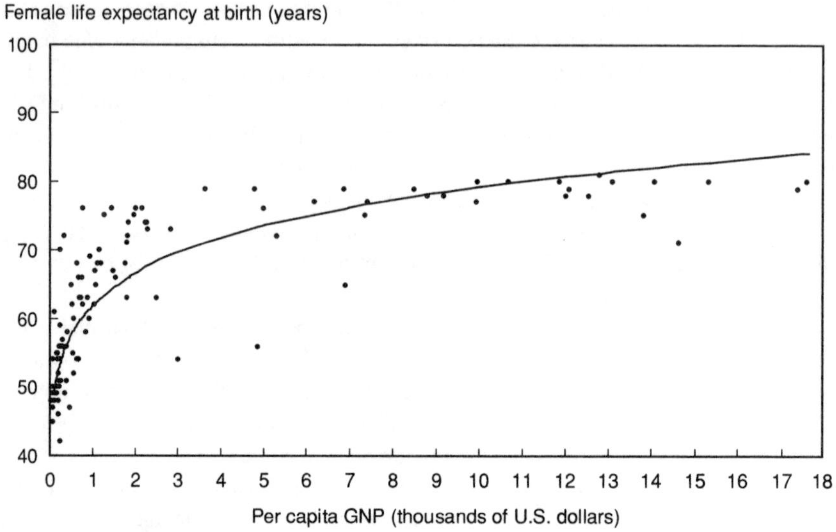

Note: The fitted line in the figure is the ordinary least-squares regression ln(female life expectancy at birth) = a + ln(GNP per capita).
Source: Appendix table A.2.

against an apparent asymptote of about 80 years.[10] Figure 2.4 shows the lower end of figure 2.3 but with two trend lines, one with and one without African countries included in the calculation.[11]

For both indicators, there appears to be a large scope for policy to have an effect. Let us assume for the moment that the trend line (with Africa in figure 2.4) has a causal interpretation. Bangladesh could expect to increase female life expectancy by five to eight years if it succeeded in doubling per capita income over the next decade. That feat would require real growth in GNP per capita of about 7 percent a year, but Bangladesh's GNP per capita has grown at an annual rate of only 0.3 percent since 1965. In contrast, by the example of China, India, Myanmar, and Sri Lanka, Bangladesh could expect, through decisions on health policy, to improve female life expectancy by 7 to more than 20 years in the same period even if income increases slowly.

Conclusion

The foregoing cross-regional and cross-country comparisons provide only a rough starting point for an analysis of the sources of improved health outcomes, particularly policy and financing. These simple aggregative statistics show that Asia, which contains over half the world's population and a large share of its poorest inhabitants, has performed well in absolute terms and relative to other developing regions in improving health and fertility indicators. Yet within Asia there are large differences in performance among countries. Although such factors as income and the physical environment are certainly important, some of the variance appears to be related to systematic differences in program effort and physical inputs.

China's experience is a particularly good example of successful policies. It achieved Bangladesh's current level of life expectancy (50 years) as early as 1968. Despite political and economic upheavals over the following decade, by 1978 life expectancy had risen to 66 years. Although China's per capita GNP also increased over the same period, there is little question that its achievement benefited directly from choices in health policy.

In contrast, several of the countries—including Bangladesh, Nepal, India, and Bhutan—that started at low levels of life expectancy in 1965 also had the smallest improvement over the following two decades, and they still rank near the bottom relative to other countries. They start the 1990s with relatively low immunization rates, small endowments of personnel, low rates of attendance by trained personnel during pregnancy and childbirth, and difficult public health problems. Improving performance in these countries may require large additions to domestic resources in the health sector, but it would also certainly require careful targeting of expenditure.

Figure 2.4 Female life expectancy at birth and per capita GNP, selected Asian countries and world trend, 1986

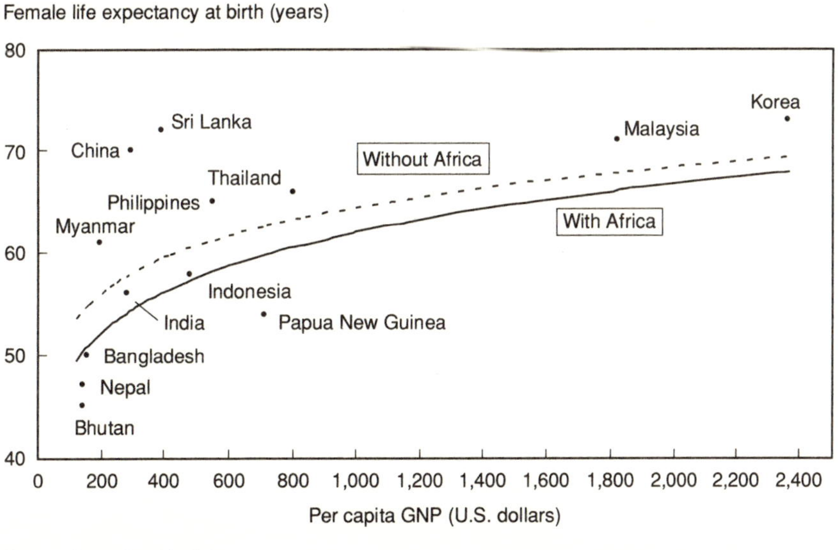

Source: Appendix table A.2.

Notes

1. The infant mortality rate is the number of infants dying before age one, per thousand live births. The child mortality rate is the proportion of youngsters alive at age one who die before their fifth birthday, per thousand one-year-olds.

2. The total fertility rate is the total number of children an average woman would bear if her experience is the same as women currently in their childbearing years.

3. Replacement fertility is the level of fertility at which women have exactly enough daughters to replace themselves, which would eventually keep the population constant. Replacement fertility is roughly two children per couple, but it technically means that a net reproduction rate of one is reached (when a fixed cohort of girls can be expected to just reproduce themselves). A population that reaches replacement fertility will continue to grow if a large proportion of women are in their childbearing years.

4. It is essential to keep in mind that immunizations do not directly affect infant mortality (except tetanus shots for the mother) because children rarely get the full series before their first birthdays. However, a program that delivers immunizations may have side benefits that affect infant mortality.

5. All dollar amounts are current U.S. dollars, unless otherwise specified.

6. However, Thailand experienced substantial improvements in infant and child mortality, suggesting that its problem lies in slow improvement in adult mortality.

7. The contraceptive prevalence rate is the proportion of all couples of childbearing age using sterilization, intrauterine devices, or oral and injectable contraceptives.

8. *Physicians* may include registered physicians and medical assistants who are less trained but perform as physicians in some areas. *Nursing personnel* includes all types of nurses, plus paraprofessional health workers, such as first aid assistants and traditional midwives who have undergone training. Unfortunately, these definitions vary across countries.

9. Many physicians in China would not be classified as such in other countries. India's nursing personnel includes many lower-level personnel.

10. Although the regression line does not recognize an upper bound!

11. Two lines are not shown in figure 2.2 because excluding Africa has an almost negligible effect.

3

Health, Demography, and Health Financing

This chapter assembles information on mortality patterns and the age structure of populations in Asia and attempts to draw from those patterns implications for health policy and health financing. Readers new to the health sector will be amazed at how little we really know about health conditions in developing countries and how feeble the data are on which policy decisions must be based. The most extensive and comparable data are available on infant mortality, which is discussed in more detail.

We have virtually no standardized information on morbidity for the Asian sample; the discussion in this chapter focuses on mortality. The health profile described in this chapter is determined by the interaction of age-specific mortality, age-specific causes of death, and the age structure of the population. Mortality and age structure are discussed separately, with conservative inferences drawn in an informal manner from overall trends in both.

There are several references to the health transition and adult mortality literatures in the following pages. The first focuses on the movement of societies from high mortality to low mortality, and the second on the relatively greater importance of adult morbidity and mortality in countries that have made this transition. Few low-income countries other than China and Sri Lanka have made this transition.

References are also made to *diseases of poverty*, a concept that has several interpretations. One interpretation particularly appropriate to low-mortality environments is that the incidence of virtually every disease is highest among the poor. Thus neoplasms (tumors) and circulatory diseases could be viewed as diseases of poverty. In low-mortality environments, both the rich and the poor tend to die of chronic diseases and accidents, but the poor tend to die earlier. If one argues that neoplasms and circulatory diseases should not have a major claim on government budgets because that would tend to favor the old and those who are financially more secure, the argument would have to address the problem that the poor also die from those diseases. On the other hand, targeting government spending to specific diseases would not be a good way to target the poor. Because ill health can reduce even a middle-class household to poverty, it has consequences for income distribution that might concern governments.

A second interpretation—the one used here—is relevant to high-mortality countries. In a high-mortality environment, poorer people tend to have a much higher probability of dying from infectious and parasitic diseases and to have extremely high infant mortality rates. And large percentages of the poor do not live long enough to die from such diseases as neoplasms and circulatory problems. Mortality rates for children age 0–5, for example, vary by residence and mother's education, which are generally good proxies for income. Mortality rates for children of women with no education are at least three times higher than for children of women with at least a seventh-grade education. This is not to say that the poor do not die of chronic diseases, of course, only that far larger percentages of people born into poor households fail to survive to the age at which symptoms of chronic diseases begin to appear. Furthermore, many of the health problems that plague the poor, especially high infant mortality (often related to diarrhea and acute respiratory infection) and infectious and parasitic diseases, are related to substandard environmental conditions and low education levels, which tend to be typical for poor populations. The concept of diseases of poverty as used in this chapter is based on the differences in the causes of death between the rich and the poor in high-mortality countries. This broad classification is not exhaustive, but it is meant to capture an important characteristic of high-mortality environments.

Mortality and health policy

Causes of death

Data that are comparable across developing countries are not available for most mortality and morbidity indicators.[1] At best, we have rough estimates across broad regions on causes of death around 1980.

Asia accounted for 58 percent of the world's population and 67 percent of worldwide deaths during the reference period in table 3.1.[2] A close look at the distribution within Asia, however, is more revealing. South Asia[3] alone accounted for 50 percent of all deaths, although it contained only 33 percent of the world's population. Deaths by certain causes are even more concentrated in South Asia. The region accounted for more than half of all deaths due to illnesses during the perinatal period (infancy), complications of pregnancy, and infectious and parasitic diseases—diseases that characterize poor, high-mortality environments. As would be expected, however, South Asia's share of deaths due to circulatory diseases and neoplasms was far smaller than its share of the world's population.

Nearly 70 percent of deaths in South Asia are caused by infectious and parasitic diseases or unknown causes, compared with only 20 percent in the more developed

Table 3.1 Deaths in Asia as a percentage of deaths in world, by cause of death, 1980

Category	*East Asia*	*South Asia*	*Asia*
Certain diseases of infancy	12	52	64
Complications of pregnancy and childbirth	18	51	69
Infectious and parasitic	12	53	65
Other and unknown	18	45	63
Injury and poisoning	24	33	57
Diseases of the circulatory system	22	24	46
Neoplasms	22	21	43
Population as percentage of world population	26	33	58
All deaths	17	50	67

Source: Hakulinen and others 1986a and 1986b.

countries (table 3.2). In East Asia, these two causes account for 44 percent of deaths, still more than double that in the more developed countries.

In general, mortality patterns in South Asia conform closely to those in less developed countries, while mortality patterns in East Asia lie between those of South Asia and more developed countries. Thus, although data on the age structure of mortality are lacking for South Asia, the aggregate pattern for less developed countries—for which data are available—provides a reasonably good guide. We can similarly assume that for East Asia, the age structure of mortality is somewhere between the patterns characterizing the more and less developed world regions. These assumptions are consistent with more recent estimates of causes of death using a data base with observations on China and India (table 3.3). For the most part, table 3.3 mimics the information in table 3.2; however, the comparison of China and India

Table 3.2 Deaths by cause in Asia and in the world, by level of development, 1980
(percent)

Disease category	*East Asia*	*South Asia*	*More developed countries*	*Less developed countries*
Certain diseases of infancy	4	8	2	8
Complications of pregnancy and childbirth	1	1	0	1
Infectious and parasitic	23	44	8	40
Other and unknown	21	23	12	23
Injury and poisoning	7	4	6	5
Diseases of the circulatory system	34	16	54	19
Neoplasms	11	4	19	6
Total	101	100	101	102

Note: Columns do not add to 100 because of rounding.
Source: Hakulinen and others 1986a and 1986b.

Table 3.3 Female deaths in Asia and in more developed countries, by cause, 1985
(percent)

Disease category	*India*	*China*	*Other developing Asian countries*	*More developed countries*
Certain diseases of infancy	11	3	7	1
Complications of pregnancy and childbirth	2	0	1	0
Infectious and parasitic	41	26	36	7
Other and unknown	25	13	26	15
Injury and poisoning	6	14	4	4
Diseases of the circulatory system	11	31	19	56
Neoplasms	4	12	7	17
Total	100	100	100	100

Source: Bulatao, Lopez, and Stevens 1989, table 2.2.

demonstrates how quickly successful health policies can change the causes of death. China, whose male life expectancy was at approximate parity with that of India in 1950, now has one about 13 years longer. This change, along with lower fertility in China, has led to China having an older population than India, with a substantially different cause-of-death structure. Despite its older population, China's crude death rate for men in 1985 was estimated to be 26 percent lower than India's.

Table 3.4 incorporates two weighting schemes into the distribution of deaths by cause (for both males and females) for poor and wealthy countries. (The first set of columns shows the unweighted distribution.) The second set of columns disregards all deaths among those over age 65. This weighting assumes that government health

Table 3.4 Distribution of deaths by cause in less developed and more developed countries, using two simple weighting schemes, 1985
(percent)

	All deaths		*Deaths under age 65*		*Years of life lost*	
Disease category	*Less developed*	*More developed*	*Less developed*	*More developed*	*Less developed*	*More developed*
Certain diseases of infancy	8	1	12	4	16	8
Complications of pregnancy and childbirth	1	0	1	0	1	0
Infectious and parasitic	36	9	42	13	46	18
Other and unknown	21	15	19	19	20	25
Injury and poisoning	8	6	10	15	9	17
Diseases of the circulatory system	19	50	11	29	6	17
Neoplasms	7	18	6	21	3	14
Total	100	99	101	101	101	99

Source: Bulatao, Lopez, and Stevens 1989, table 2.8.

policy should be concerned with premature death, on the assumption that all deaths over 65 occur near the end of a normal life. This approach increases the weight given to deaths in infancy and those due to infectious and parasitic diseases, and substantially reduces the weight of circulatory diseases in the table. The third set of columns gives the percentage distribution of potential years of life lost due to each disease category, which adds more weight to diseases that kill the young. (It is a simple calculation that assumes life expectancy is 75 years for everyone and that death occurs at the mean age for each age group; see Bulatao, Lopez, and Stevens 1989.) This weighting gives value to government policy that aims to maximize total years of life for the society. The approach weights diseases of infancy and deaths due to infectious and parasitic diseases even more heavily relative to deaths from circulatory diseases and neoplasms. A third alternative is to weight years of life lost by lost earnings. This approach would tend to increase the relative weight given to neoplasms and circulatory diseases to the extent that they strike people in their years of peak earnings. However, the theme is clear. There is little question that infectious and parasitic diseases merit continued attention in developing countries. This statement is accurate for Southeast Asia and doubly true for South Asia. Health policies that favor improved health among the young relative to the old would commensurately weight infectious and parasitic diseases more heavily.

Age structure of mortality

Death rates in all groups in the less developed countries exceed those in the more developed countries, but the largest differential occurs in the youngest age group (table 3.5). The 0–14 age group suffers seven times as many deaths per thousand in the less developed countries as in the more developed countries. Although the 15–44 age group has a low death rate in the less developed countries, it is about three times that in the more developed countries. The death rate in the 45–64 age group is about twice as high in the poorer countries.

In the less developed countries, 71 percent of the deaths in the youngest group are due either to problems at or near birth, or to infectious and parasitic diseases. Most of the remaining deaths result from unknown causes. Although fewer children die in more developed countries, they tend to die from the same three causes (although the distribution among the three is different), which account for 85 percent of the deaths.

Death rates for the older age groups are similar across levels of development, but, as is clear from table 3.5, it is in this age group that distinctive differences in causes of death arise. Infectious and parasitic diseases cause nearly half the deaths among those age 15–44 in the less developed countries, but they cause less than a tenth of deaths for that group in the more developed countries. People in this age group in developing countries are most likely to die from problems of pregnancy, infectious and parasitic diseases, and unknown causes, while those in the same age group in developed countries are most likely to die from injuries, circulatory diseases, and tumors. These differences in causes of death persist into the 45–64 age group.

Table 3.5 Age structure of mortality by cause for more developed and less developed world regions, 1980
(percent, except death rate)

	Ages 0–14		*Ages 15–44*		*Ages 45–64*	
Disease category	*Less developed*	*More developed*	*Less developed*	*More developed*	*Less developed*	*More developed*
Certain diseases of infancy	17	31				
Complications of pregnancy and childbirth			4	1		
Infectious and parasitic	54	26	44	7	29	5
Other and unknown	24	28	17	13	19	9
Injury and poisoning	3	10	16	41	5	7
Diseases of the circulatory system	2	3	14	23	34	48
Neoplasms	0	3	6	17	14	32
Total	100	101	101	102	101	101
Death rate (per thousand)	13.9	2.1	3.8	1.4	16.9	8.5

Note: The less developed and more developed regions in the table are those used by the U.N. classification system. Data do not add up to 100 because of rounding.
Source: Hakulinen and others 1986a and 1986b.

Although the proportion of older people in less developed countries dying of chronic diseases rises to nearly half, about a third die of infectious and parasitic diseases.

One other feature of these mortality differentials is worth noting. Figures 3.1 through 3.3 display crude death rates by cause for the three age groups and for three levels of development. These figures, which share the same scale, show vividly that death preys disproportionately on the young in developing countries. What most distinguishes the pattern of mortality across age groups in less developed and least developed countries from that in more developed countries are the extremely high toll taken by infectious and parasitic diseases and the large number of deaths in the other and unknown category. In contrast, differences in death rates across levels of development for injuries and poisonings, circulatory diseases, and neoplasms are small. Death rates in the poorer countries exceed those in the developed countries for every disease category and every age group, except for neoplasms in the oldest group (figure 3.3). The major distinguishing feature of even adult mortality in the developing country sample is the prevalence of infectious and parasitic diseases as a cause of death.

The special issue of maternal mortality in South Asia

In 1947 life expectancy in Sri Lanka was 44; it rose to 58 in 1954, to 62 in 1965, and to 65 in 1972. Age- and sex-specific death rates are shown for Sri Lanka for the mid-1940s and the early 1970s in figure 3.4, which is on a logarithmic scale that com-

Figure 3.1 Death rates for ages 0-14, by level of development, around 1980

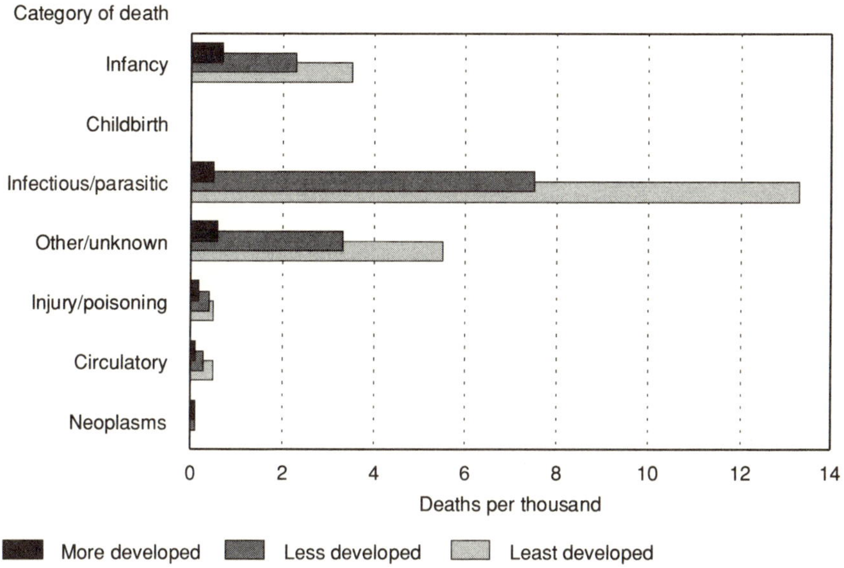

Source: Hakulinen and others 1986.

Figure 3.2 Death rates for ages 15-44, by level of development, around 1980

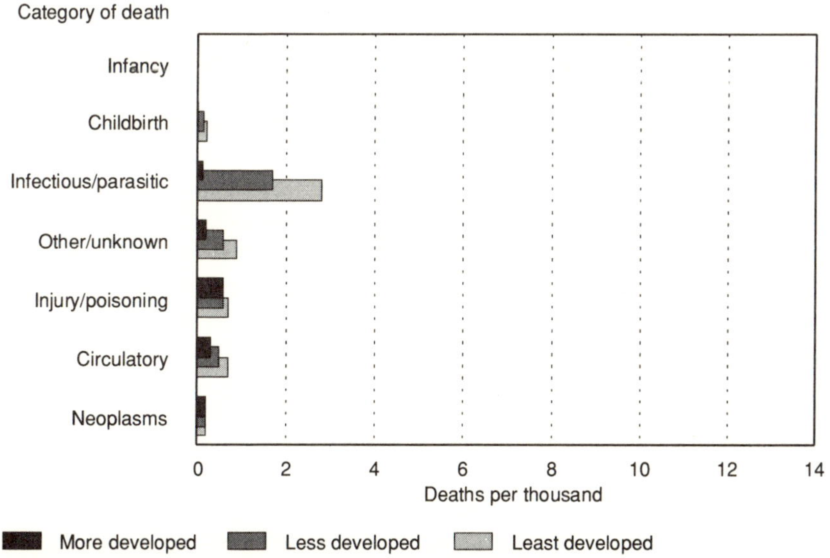

Source: Hakulinen and others 1986.

Figure 3.3 Death rates for ages 45-64, by level of development, around 1980

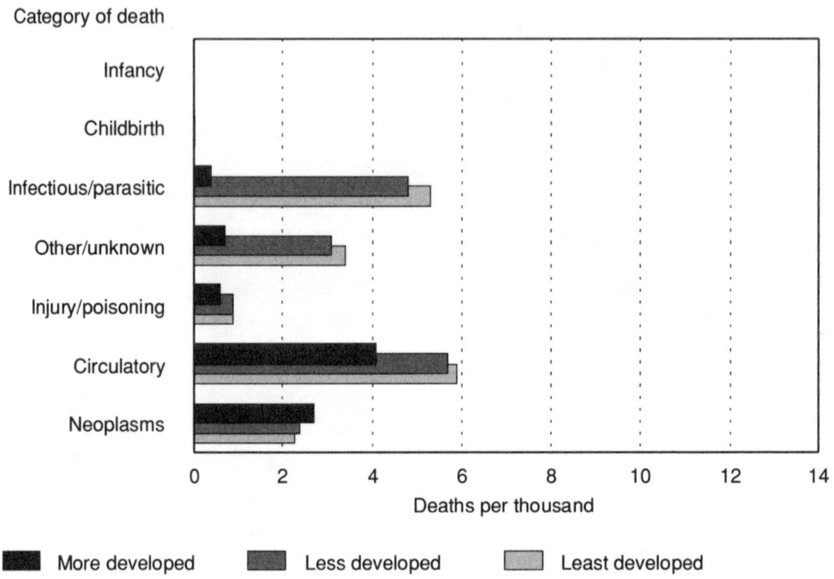

Source: Hakulinen and others 1986.

presses the y-axis and allows a larger range of numbers to be seen. Across the two time periods, mortality at every age declined—the broken lines for 1970–72 are lower than the solid lines for 1945–47. Although the largest absolute changes were in infant mortality, a second notable change was the reduction in death rates for women during their childbearing years. In 1945–47, female death rates exceeded male death rates from birth, with a widening gap after age 10 that persisted through the childbearing years. The death rate for men began to exceed that for women after age 40. Although the increased risk for women between ages 10 and 40 is still evident in 1970–72, by that time it was greatly reduced, and death rates for men actually exceeded those for women at every age after puberty. Sri Lanka's progress in health has been closely connected with the reduction in the risk of death for females during the childbearing years and the associated reduction in the risk of death for infants.

Bangladesh's current male and female age-specific death rates (figure 3.5) are similar to India's and to Nepal's, which are not shown. Sex-specific death rates in Bangladesh in 1981 were very similar to those for Sri Lanka in 1947. Death rates for women of childbearing age in Bangladesh in 1981 were so high that they exceeded those for men in the same age group 16 years earlier (in 1965), despite improvements in overall life expectancy. Bangladesh has not only started much later than Sri Lanka in reducing mortality, but it has also shown significantly slower progress and has made little headway in reducing the dangers associated with childbirth.

Mortality patterns in the Philippines (figure 3.6) are similar to profiles for Hong Kong, Korea, Malaysia, Singapore, and Thailand. The childbearing "hump" in mortality for women is almost nonexistent. The female death rate never rises above the male death rate, unlike in the South Asian countries.

More recent data for India are shown in figures 3.7 and 3.8. Chatterjee (1990) finds that India's average life expectancy for females has increased to about equal that for males during the past decade, but the gains have come at ages above 35 years and have not affected women in their childbearing years. The same mortality hump that shows up for women during the childbearing years for Sri Lanka in the 1940s and Bangladesh in 1981 plagued women in urban and rural India in 1984 (figures 3.7 and 3.8). But the difference in mortality rates is not confined to the childbearing years, although it increases over that period. Chatterjee suggests that the mortality differential is tied to the relative economic value of women in the household and cites evidence that survival rates vary inversely with the size of dowry (where larger dowries are common, women represent a greater drain on the family) and directly with female labor force participation. There is also some evidence that female survival rates are higher among households with smaller landholdings, where women's economic contributions are more highly valued.

Figure 3.4 Age-specific death rates, by sex, Sri Lanka, 1945-47 and 1970-72

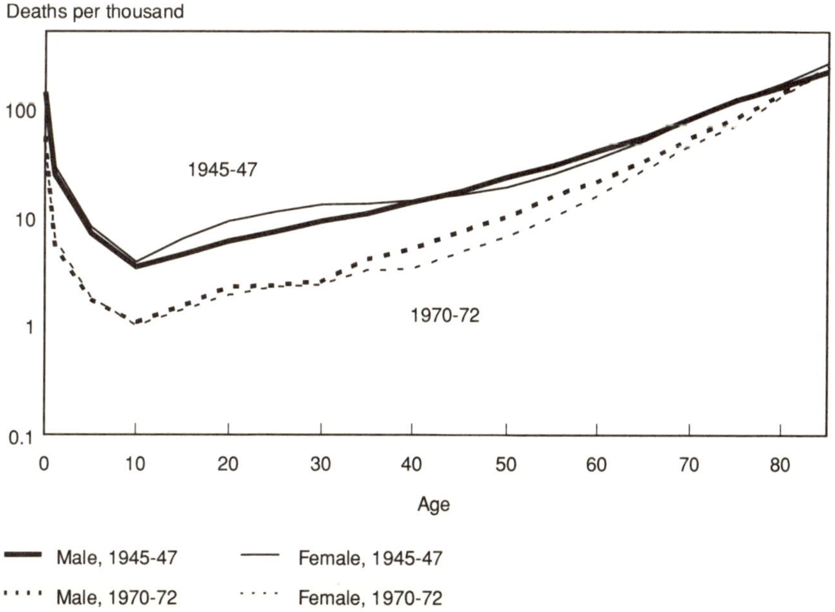

Source: United Nations 1986.

Figure 3.5 Age-specific death rates, by sex, Bangladesh, 1964-65 and 1981

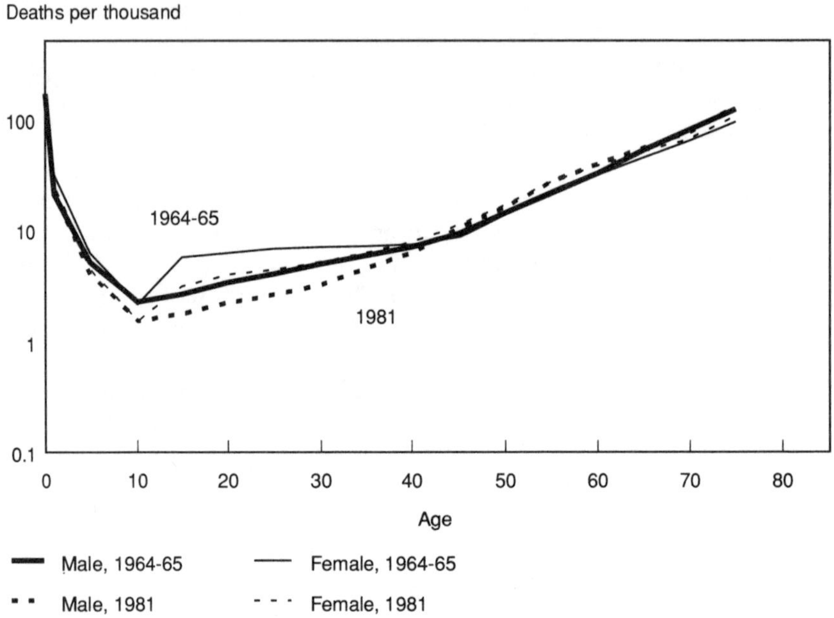

Source: United Nations 1986.

The transition to better health and higher survival rates for women in South Asia is dependent on changes in prenatal care, birth practices, tetanus immunizations, nutrition, the number of babies born to a woman, resource allocations within the home, and other variables. Many of these factors can be affected by health policies. For a large share of the population in South Asia, the differences in mortality between males and females, coupled with continued high infant mortality, provide a clear focus for health (and, of course, population) policies. This is not new information. Health and population policy statements in South Asia recognize the importance of these problems, which almost certainly arise from behavior and from resource allocations in the home. However, a question raised by these figures is to what extent government allocations reinforce or counteract the domestic behavior that leads to relatively high death rates for young girls and for women during their childbearing years.

Summary

An important difference between high- and low-mortality countries is the age and sex profile of mortality. For the countries with a short life expectancy, improvements will be tied closely to success in reducing infant mortality and eliminating the mor-

Figure 3.6 Age-specific death rates, by sex, Philippines, 1969-71

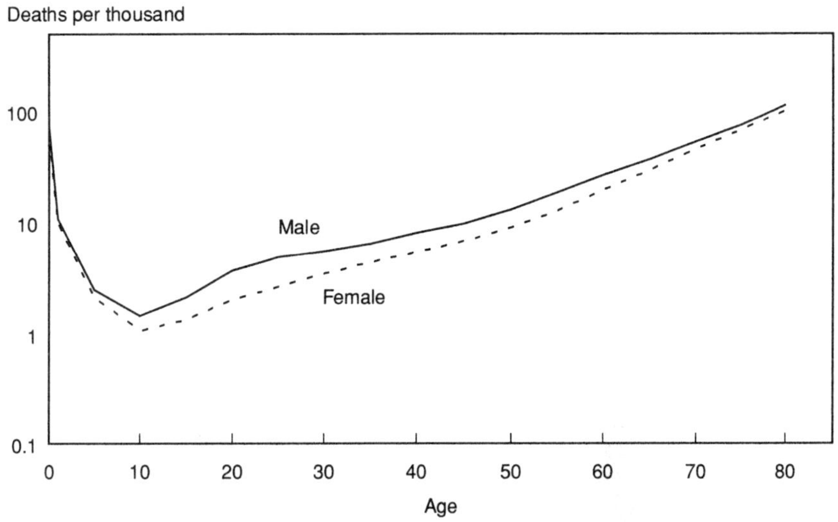

Source: United Nations 1986.

Figure 3.7 Age-specific death rates, by sex, rural India, 1984

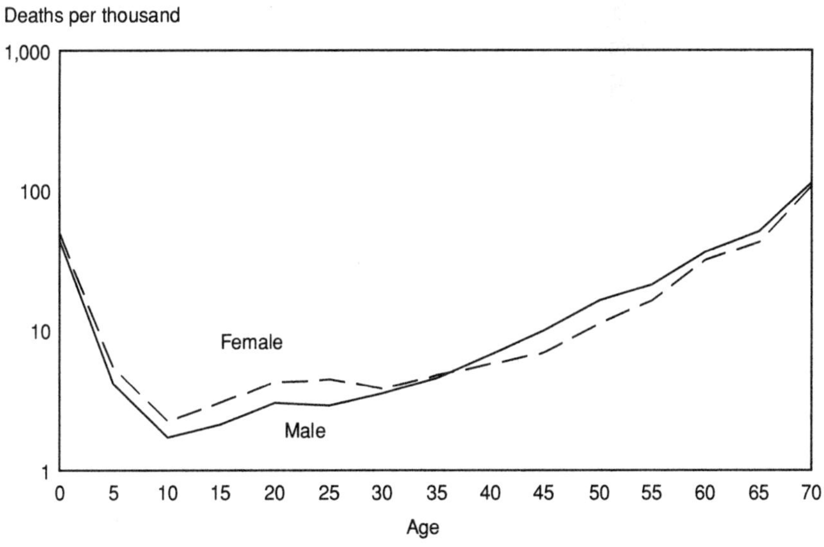

Source: Chatterjee 1990.

Figure 3.8 Age-specific death rates, by sex, urban India, 1984

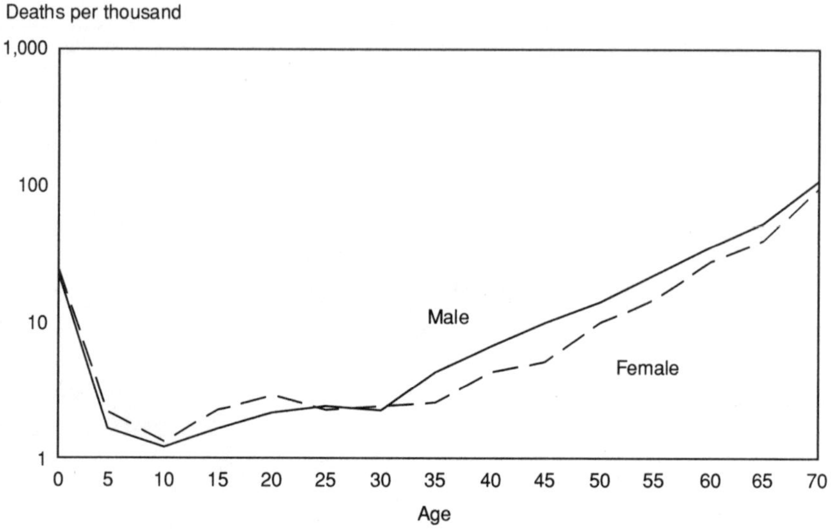

Source: Chatterjee 1990.

tality differential for women during their childbearing years. These data largely confirm the assumptions that have driven donor and government planning in the health sector during the last 15 years—that the mortality problems of developing countries are tied to infectious and parasitic diseases and to childbirth. However, the data make clearer exactly what the effects of reducing the incidence of these diseases will be. Targeting childbirth will tend to improve outcomes for two important groups: it will reduce the huge differentials in mortality rates for the youngest children (raising life expectancy almost in lockstep with reductions in infant mortality), and it will reduce the risk of death for women in the 15–44 age group. Targeting infectious and parasitic diseases will reinforce that effect in the younger age groups and reduce death rates in all age groups.

It is somewhat surprising to find that reducing the incidence of infectious and parasitic diseases appears to be so important even for the 14–44 and 45–64 age groups. Some analysts have begun to argue that greater attention to chronic diseases is necessary because of the aging of populations in developing countries. While the evidence cited in this paper is derived from aggregate statistics and will not necessarily hold for specific countries, it suggests that reducing deaths from infectious and parasitic diseases among older groups will be nearly enough to push them to the life expectancy levels achieved in the wealthier countries.

From a financing standpoint, this finding highlights the interaction between policy choices on how to pay for health care and the proper role of the government in financing specific types of health activities. Interventions that reduce infectious and parasitic diseases usually have benefits that extend beyond the individual and therefore merit subsidization by the government on grounds of pure economic efficiency. In contrast, the treatment of chronic diseases tends to be of a catastrophic, individual-oriented nature. Arguments for government subsidies for curative services must generally be made on grounds other than economic efficiency. From a standpoint of economic efficiency, there is consequently a hierarchy of activities when assigning responsibility to governments. Ranking high among them are activities to combat the causes of death dominating developing country mortality profiles.[4]

For the sample of Asian countries that is our focus, there are no comparable data available on disease incidence, mortality, or morbidity. In the absence of such data, an overall assessment of the major health problems by national health administrators provides an idea of the primary disease problems (table 3.6). Diseases that were cited for at least four countries, shaded in table 3.6, include circulatory diseases, diarrhea, gastrointestinal problems, infections, leprosy, malaria, malnutrition, respiratory conditions, and tuberculosis. It is almost conventional wisdom that public health interventions exist that can prevent or delay most of these diseases, including circulatory diseases,[5] and that most of the diseases are identified as much with poverty and human behavior as with the specific disease agents that cause them. Malaria—almost a pure public health problem in an economic sense—was the most frequently cited health problem, mentioned by every country administrator but those from Korea and Malaysia. Box 3.1 contains a more detailed discussion of the prevalence of these diseases.

Hansluwka (1986a) has summarized these patterns in terms of population. Almost 1,200 million Asians (primarily Chinese and Japanese) live in countries that have completed the transition to low-mortality societies, most within a single generation. Another 150 million Asians live where health conditions are improving swiftly, in countries with a mix of health problems. These countries are in Southeast Asia for the most part. However, nearly half the population (1,130 million) lives in countries where progress over the last 30 years has been slow. These countries, which have fallen far behind their neighbors, are primarily in South Asia (not including Sri Lanka). But even in countries that have, on the whole, performed well, significant proportions of the population have not kept up. This is particularly true in China.

Demography and health policy

Coupled with age-specific cause-of-death patterns, the age structure of the population largely determines a country's mortality profile. Although concern has been expressed by some about changing health needs in Asia due to the aging of the population, overall demographic changes actually point to healthier populations over the next 15 years. Table 3.7 shows changes in the age structure of the countries in the Asian sample between 1990 and 2005, which is a reasonable planning horizon for both capital and personnel investments.[6]

Table 3.6 Major health problems in Asia, mid-1970s and mid-1980s

Health problem	*Bangladesh*	*India*	*Indonesia*	*Korea*	*Malaysia*	*Myanmar*	*Nepal*	*Papua New Guinea*	*Philippines*	*Sri Lanka*	*Thailand*
Accidents				3	•						1
Cholera			•								
Cardiovascular				2	1	1					
Circulatory			3	1	1				1		2
Diarrhea	•		2					•			3
Diphtheria											•
Drug abuse									•		
Gastrointestinal	1					3	•			•	
Infectious diseases		•	•				1			1	
Leprosy	•	3				•				•	•
Malaria	•	1	•			•	•	2	•	•	•
Malnutrition						•			•	•	•
Measles							•				
Meningitis								•			
Neoplasms				•	2			•			
Nervous system							3				
Parasitic							1			1	
Perinatal								3		3	
Pneumonia						2		1			
Pollution				•							
Pyrexia	3										
Respiratory	2		1		3		2			2	
Sanitation									•		
Schistosomiasis									•		
Tuberculosis	•	2	•		•	•	•	•			
Venereal					•					•	
Whooping cough											•

Note: • denotes problems cited by health administrators in 1975. Numbers refer to rankings of problems as cited by health administrators in a 1985 evaluation of Health for All by the Year 2000, a World Health Organization-sponsored goal for the health sector in developing countries. A repeat of the same number for a country denotes a tie. Shaded diseases were cited by administrators of at least four countries.
Source: Hansluwka 1986b, and United Nations 1986.

Table 3.7 Change in size of each cohort in selected Asian countries, 1990–2005
(percent)

		Age group				
Country	*Sex*	*0–14*	*15–44*	*45–64*	*65+*	*Total*
Bangladesh	Male	16	52	43	35	35
	Female	15	50	62	47	36
	Total	16	51	52	41	36
China	Male	15	7	51	58	19
	Female	17	8	58	52	21
	Total	16	8	55	55	20
India	Male	3	40	36	53	26
	Female	3	39	45	56	27
	Total	3	40	40	55	26
Indonesia	Male	5	40	41	67	28
	Female	5	36	45	73	27
	Total	5	38	43	70	28
Korea	Male	5	8	57	85	18
	Female	5	10	50	80	19
	Total	5	9	54	82	18
Malaysia	Male	-3	34	82	58	27
	Female	-2	33	81	72	28
	Total	-3	33	81	65	27
Myanmar	Male	16	31	66	37	30
	Female	15	30	65	35	30
	Total	16	31	66	36	30
Nepal	Male	43	54	39	52	48
	Female	45	52	25	75	46
	Total	44	53	32	64	47
Papua New Guinea	Male	22	43	40	65	35
	Female	24	45	49	90	38
	Total	23	44	45	77	37
Philippines	Male	9	40	83	69	33
	Female	9	41	80	74	34
	Total	9	40	81	72	34
Sri Lanka	Male	1	28	42	49	22
	Female	2	25	60	79	25
	Total	1	27	51	63	24
Thailand	Male	0	24	68	72	23
	Female	0	24	64	77	24
	Total	0	24	66	75	23

Source: Zachariah and Vu 1988.

An important change masked by the size of the intervals chosen for table 3.7 is an actual drop in the size of the 0–4 age group for most countries between 1990 and 2005. Table 3.8 shows projected changes in the size of that group over the period. By 2005, 88 percent of Asia's population will live in countries with fewer toddlers than

Box 3.1 Epidemiological situation in Asia, mid-1980s

A recent assessment of the epidemiological situation in Asia (Hansluwka 1986b) identified the following health problems:

Malaria. In South Asia, 96 percent of the population of 877 million is exposed to malaria risk. Except for in a small area of Nepal, malaria control operations are taking place. In East Asia and Oceania, 80 percent of the population of 1,653 million live in originally malarious areas, but malaria has been eradicated in areas where 15 percent live and creates only limited risk for 26 percent of the population. Hong Kong, Korea, Singapore, and large areas of China are considered to be free of malaria. A 1984 assessment found that malaria was well controlled in China and Malaysia; in Bangladesh and Indonesia there was an improvement; in India, Myanmar, and Papua New Guinea the situation was stable; in Nepal, the Philippines, Sri Lanka, and Thailand there was an increase.

Malnutrition. In Southeast Asia, low birth weight was estimated to be a problem in 30 percent of the births; protein-energy malnutrition affected 60 percent of children 0–5 years old; and anemia afflicted 59 percent of the women between 15 and 49 years of age. Per capita calorie supply in 1980 was below the estimated requirement in Bangladesh, India, and Papua New Guinea.

Leprosy. The incidence of leprosy seems to have increased in Southeast Asia, but there are serious problems with reporting systems.

Diarrhea. This continues to be a major threat to infants and children.

Environment. Almost all countries in the region improved coverage of safe rural water supply systems between 1975 and 1983, but Bangladesh and Papua New Guinea appear to have fallen behind. The situation is much worse for urban water supply, with some improvement in Bangladesh and Myanmar but either no change (at less than complete coverage) or a worsening of coverage in the rest of the countries. The situation is similar for sanitation, with some improvement in rural areas and a deterioration in urban areas. In rural areas of Bangladesh, India, and Nepal, improvement has stalled at near-zero levels of coverage.

Vaccine-preventable diseases. As seen earlier, in most countries there has been a vast improvement reported in the incidence of diseases that can be prevented by vaccines, although in many it is from very low levels.

there are today. The 5–14 age group in most countries will, however, show a small increase. The 15–44 age group will grow by over 25 percent in every country but China and Korea, and all countries will experience growth of more than 30 percent in the 45–64 age group. About half the countries will show increases exceeding 50 percent in that age group. Growth in the group of those older than 65 will exceed 30 percent in all countries but will be 70 percent or more in over half the countries.

These changes in the age structure of the population are reflected in changes in the crude death rate, which is shown in figure 3.9 for 1990 and 2005.[7] Crude death rates are heavily influenced not only by health conditions but also by the age structure of the population, so that they tend to rise as a population ages. In only China and Korea

Table 3.8 Change in size of 0–4 age group in selected Asian countries, 1990–2005
(percent)

Negative		*Positive*		*High*	
China	-3	Korea	3	Bangladesh	11
India	-3	Philippines	4	Myanmar	9
Indonesia	-1	Nepal	33		
Malaysia	-13	Papua New Guinea	18		
Sri Lanka	-9				
Thailand	-6				

Source: Zachariah and Vu 1988.

is the crude death rate projected to begin increasing over the next 15 years (in Sri Lanka the rate will remain unchanged), which reflects success in reducing both birthrates and death rates over the last two decades. China and Korea have already begun undergoing substantial changes in patterns of mortality and morbidity. For the

Figure 3.9 Crude death rates in selected Asian countries and the United States, 1990 and 2005

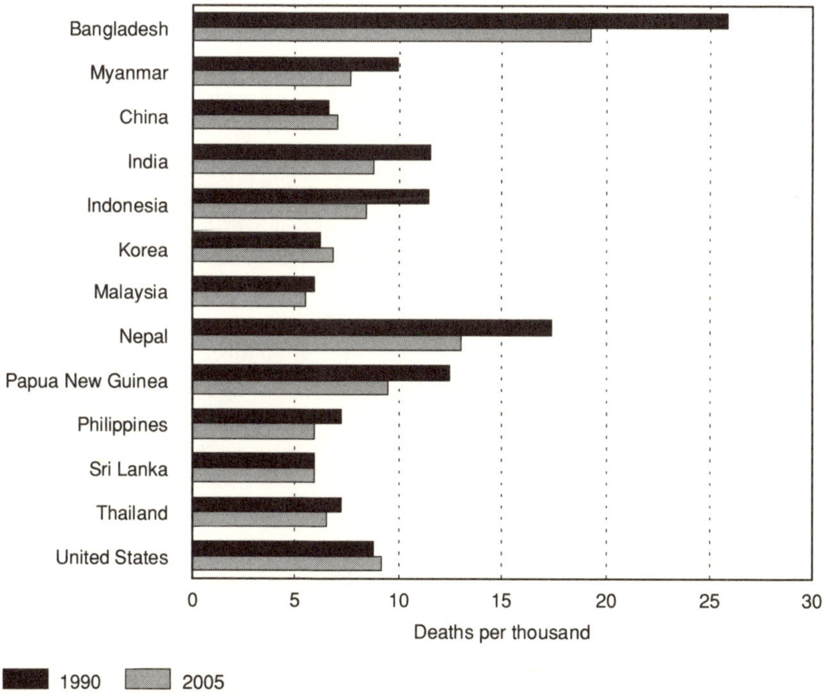

Source: Zachariah and Vu 1988.

rest of the sample, however, this transition will be slower; in fact, the outlook is bright. They will have fewer deaths per thousand because their populations will be concentrated in the healthier age groups.

The large percentage increases of the oldest groups have caused concern that the incidence of chronic diseases will increase rapidly. The fear is that these demographic changes will contribute to the two-tier morbidity and mortality structures already emerging in some countries, where there is continued high incidence of diseases connected with high mortality, especially in rural areas, but with an accompanying increase in chronic health problems, primarily in urban areas.

While chronic disease will become more important, in most of the sample that problem is on the horizon, not close at hand. Although the highest percentage growth rates will occur in the oldest age groups, that is primarily because the changes are taking place from a relatively low base. Figure 3.10 shows that, except in China and Korea, well over 75 percent of the population will still be under 45 in 2005. As explained above, the youngest age group will be contracting as a share of the total, as the current bulge of youngsters moves into the most productive and healthiest range of ages. The oldest two groups will grow but will remain a small share of the total population in most of the countries.

The financing issue posed by these demographic changes will be to develop institutions to make sure that the health needs of the aged can be paid for either by themselves when they eventually need care or through social insurance that shares costs across generations. The medical and health policy challenges lie in the future, and China and Korea (with Sri Lanka and Malaysia not far behind) have already begun to lead the way in facing those challenges. As will be discussed later, those countries are increasing health expenditure and erecting financing mechanisms to reduce health risks caused by hospitalizations. For the rest of the sample, there is time to lay the groundwork for health-financing mechanisms that will provide the means to pay for the future disease burdens in an equitable and efficient manner.

Where is the immediate challenge embedded in these demographic changes? Interestingly, other than the aged, the largest and fastest growing group with clearly identifiable age-related health needs will be women of childbearing age. Except in the low-mortality countries, this group will increase its share of the population to nearly a quarter of the total over 1990–2005. These women will have fewer children, they will be more urbanized, they will have more education, and they will use more health services than were available to their mothers. They are the main group to benefit from family planning. About half the women in that cohort are now school-age children, and one of the most effective health interventions they or their future children will ever receive is being provided through their schools. The investments being made in these young women today and the services they use during their childbearing years will strongly affect the health of the 25 to 40 percent of the population under 15 in 2005.

It bears repeating that if the poorer countries in this sample can reduce deaths due to infectious diseases and other or unknown causes in the 15–64 age groups, death rates in those groups will fall very close to levels achieved in industrial countries even if chronic disease problems receive little attention. Moreover, reducing those diseases will have payoffs across the age spectrum that will not be captured by a single group.

Figure 3.10 Age structure in selected Asian countries and the United States, 1990 and 2005

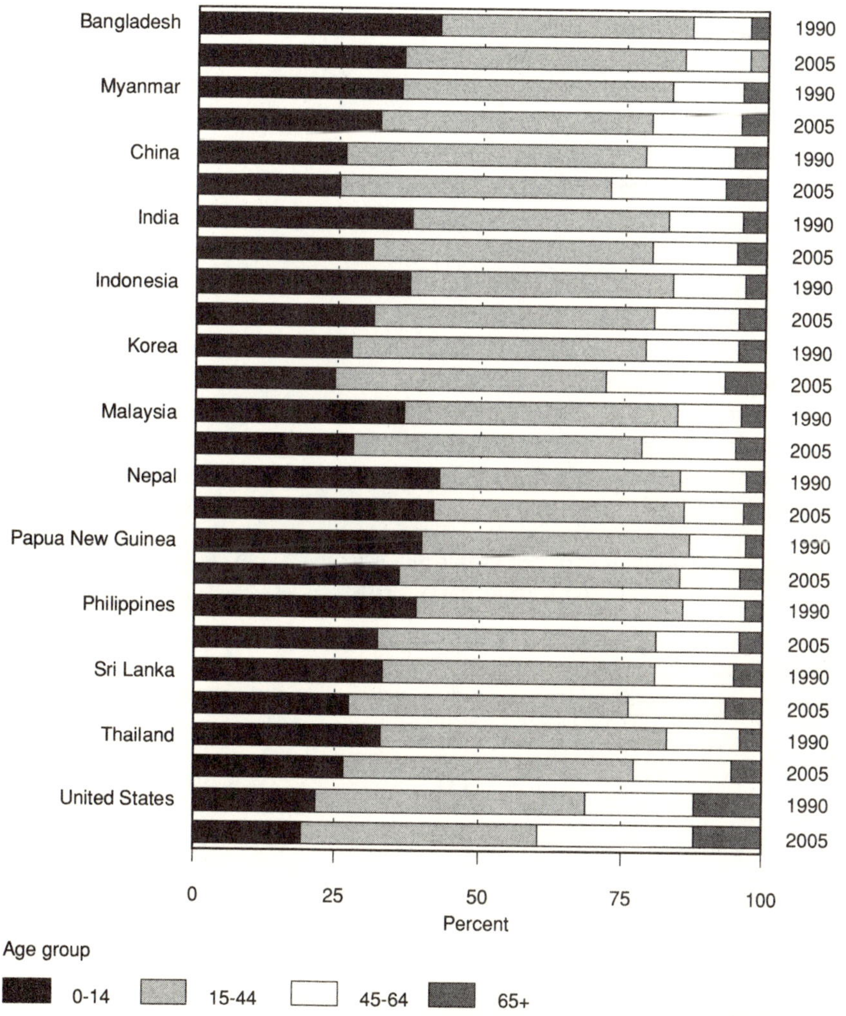

Source: Zachariah and Vu 1988.

Potential of policy to affect health: Infant mortality and health inputs

Evidence from the World Fertility Surveys: Infant mortality by residence and education

If these aggregative comparisons are accurate, the main disease problems for most of the Asian countries, especially for those with the greatest health problems, remain much the same as for the poorer countries of the world in general. The important diseases to target are infectious and parasitic; the important groups to target in most of the sample are women of childbearing age and their children. This section reviews recent systematic evidence on infant and child mortality across countries in Asia. That information, which is already quite dated, is supplemented with more recent data from Sri Lanka, Thailand, and China that provide some descriptive information on the role of the health sector in mother and child health care.

The World Fertility Surveys from the mid to late 1970s, the Contraceptive Prevalence Surveys from the early 1980s, and the Demographic and Health Surveys that are just now being published provide a wealth of household-level descriptive information on changes in fertility and child health. Data on mortality rates per thousand children between ages 0 and 5 from the World Fertility Surveys are shown in table 3.9. These numbers are generally quite high, but they refer to a period about 20 years ago. They show two distinct patterns: first, the expected pattern within countries of higher mortality in rural areas and for children of less educated women; and second, an interesting cross-national pattern. In high-mortality countries, such as Bangladesh or Nepal, the mortality rates for children of the most highly educated women are

Table 3.9 Mortality of children under 5 in selected Asian countries, by residence and mother's education, early 1970s
(deaths per thousand)

		Residence			*Mother's education*			
Country	*All children under 5*	*Metro-politan*	*Other urban*	*Rural*	*None*	*Grade 1–3*	*Grade 4–6*	*Grade 7+*
Bangladesh	215	180	188	218	222	198	186	122
Indonesia	180	143	137	188	193	194	143	77
Korea	83	63	87	90	107	94	74	56
Malaysia	61	42	46	68	67	64	56	18
Nepal	259	..	145	262	261	204	157	136
Philippines	90	57	77	98	130	118	94	53
Sri Lanka	84	71	74	87	104	97	80	55
Thailand	116	57	83	122	145	105	110	38

.. Not available.
Source: Hobcraft, McDonald, and Rutstein 1985.

Table 3.10 Mortality rates by child's age, mother's education, and residence, in Sri Lanka and Thailand, 1980–85
(per thousand)

	Sri Lanka			Thailand		
Category	*0–12 months*	*1–4 years*	*0–5 years*	*0–12 months*	*1–4 years*	*0–5 years*
By residence						
Metropolitan	33	7	39	..	..	..
Other urban	37	4	41	27	8	35
Rural	30	10	40	41	12	52
Estates	58	17	73	..	..	..
By mother's education						
None	52	20	71	54	22	74
Primary	34	9	43	39	10	49
Secondary	32	9	41	19	2	21
More	20	7	26	..	..	..
Total sample						
1980–85	32	10	42	38	11	49
1970–75	60	28	86	65	28	91
Change (percent)	-47	-64	-51	-42	-61	-46

.. Not available.
Note: Secondary for Thailand means secondary education or higher.
Source: Chayovan, Kamnuansilpa, and Knodel 1988, and Institute for Resource Development, Westinghouse, and Sri Lanka 1988.

higher than those for children of the least educated women in the countries with low child mortality rates. So, while education and residence matter, there are large differences across countries that cannot be explained by those variables. Even countries at similar overall levels of child mortality, such as Korea, the Philippines, and Sri Lanka, have different patterns across residential and educational groups.

Evidence from the Demographic and Health Surveys: 1980–85

Such cross-national comparisons of mortality patterns for the last decade will not be possible for several more years. But data from the Demographic and Health Surveys for Sri Lanka and Thailand are now available, and they provide further evidence on some of these patterns (table 3.10). Both countries have cut the death rate for children (or the probability of death from age 0 to 5) by about half since the early 1970s (table 3.9): Sri Lanka by 51 percent, Thailand by 46 percent.[8] Given the precision of these numbers, both the level and the trend in the two countries should be taken to be about the same. But large differences between rural and urban areas persist in Thailand, where infant mortality rates are actually lower in cities than in Sri Lanka. In Sri

Table 3.11 Mothers using various health inputs, by educational status, in Sri Lanka and Thailand, 1985
(percent)

	Sri Lanka				*Thailand*			
Health care input	*No education*	*Primary*	*Secondary*	*Higher than secondary*	*No education*	*Primary*	*Secondary*	*Higher than secondary*
Prenatal care (any visit)	87	96	98	99	48	78	94	100
Tetanus (1 or 2 doses)	80	79	84	86	..	..	..	..
Delivery (trained attendant)	80	92	96	99	44	64	94	99
Health card (for child age 1–2)	66	79	85	87	16	34	58	58
DPT 3 (if health card)	90	87	95	99	..	82	83	94
At least one immunization	..	..	..	..	75	89	98	100

.. Not available.

Note: Tetanus toxoid coverage not reported for Thailand. "At least one immunization" not reported for Sri Lanka.

Source: Chayovan, Kamnuansilpa, and Knodel 1988, and Institute for Resource Development, Westinghouse, and Sri Lanka 1988.

Lanka, however, child death rates are nearly the same in urban and rural areas.[9] Even so, Sri Lanka continues to have a serious problem in the poor estate sector, where child mortality is nearly 42 percent higher than the national average.

The concordance between the two countries in child mortality rates by mother's education is impressive. The mortality differential between children of women with no education and those of women with a primary education is 1.7 in Sri Lanka and 1.5 in Thailand. It is somewhat disturbing to see that whether or not mothers get some schooling has such a large effect on child mortality even after it has fallen by so much. Furthermore, in both countries there is considerably more variation in mortality rates for children age 1–4 years than in those for children age 0–12 months.

Can we detect differences in the use of health services that might contribute to these patterns across residential and educational groups? Table 3.11 shows the use of health inputs related to infant and child health by mothers according to their education for the two countries. In Sri Lanka, there are some differences across education levels in the use of health services, but at least 79 percent of all groups used prenatal care and delivery services. In Thailand, however, less than half the uneducated women used prenatal or delivery services. Substantial increases in the use of these inputs should be possible, especially among women with a primary education or less. If these inputs matter, and we assume that they do, continued gains in infant and child mortality should still be possible in Thailand through the health system, while Sri Lanka may have reached a point of sharply diminishing returns to additional health system inputs.

China's 1985 fertility survey

It may also be valuable briefly to review China's recent experience. Preliminary results from the first phase of its in-depth fertility survey are presented in table 3.12 for the three provinces that it covered. The final row of the table contains infant mortality statistics. At 15 per thousand live births, infant mortality in Shanghai is extraordinarily low, less than half that in Colombo, Sri Lanka. Hebei's infant mortality rate matches Sri Lanka's, and Shaanxi's rate is close to that of the Philippines. Although these rates are quite low by developing country standards, the variability across regions is substantial.

Shanghai proper is characterized by nearly 100 percent rates of use for each type of health system input, although rates are slightly lower in surrounding areas. In contrast, the extremely low mortality rates in the two more agricultural provinces have been achieved with rates of use of health inputs that are quite low, in most cases lower than those observed in Thailand for mothers with no education. For example, in Shaanxi, only 32 percent of the rural sample gave birth with a trained attendant present, and only 43 percent had a prenatal visit. Childbirth has somehow been made much safer without substantially greater direct use of health inputs in these two provinces. It could be caused by many unobservable factors—for example, differences in behavior, a better environment, better diets, targeting of the little health care that is

Table 3.12 Mothers using various health inputs, by urban or rural residence, in three provinces of China, 1985
(percent)

	Shaanxi (well-developed northwest province)		*Hebei (well-developed northern province)*		*Shanghai (China's largest city)*	
Health care input	*Urban (11%)*	*Rural (79%)*	*Urban (17%)*	*Rural (83%)*	*Urban (59%)*	*Rural (41%)*
Prenatal care (any visit)	80	43	73	49	98	91
Delivery by trained attendant	70	20	50	36	100	96
Delivery in hospital or clinic	54	12	40	12	100	79
Some immunization in first six months	75	43	61	58	98	93
Infant mortality rate for province	49		33		15	

Note: Infant mortality is not reported by urban/rural classification. The survey was conducted during April 1985. "Delivery in hospital or clinic" is a subset of "delivery by trained attendant."
Source: China 1986.

used to high-risk cases, or effective health education. Understanding why Hebei's infant mortality rate is lower than Thailand's despite less apparent use of medical inputs would be important for health policy.

Causes of death among children

Finally, what kills children, and can health care's effectiveness in preventing their deaths be increased? The aggregate data discussed at the beginning of the chapter outlines broad categories for causes of death, but does a finer focus provide additional information?

Table 3.13 Infant and child mortality by cause in Myanmar
(percent)

	Infant mortality		*Child mortality (in hospitals)*	
Cause of death	*In towns 1980*	*In hospitals 1982*	*Ages 1–4 1982*	*Ages 5–14 1982*
Ill-defined/other	27	23	25	34
Acute respiratory infection	14	31	26	16
Intestinal infection	10	12	26	8
Other infections	16			
Perinatal	26	22		
Tetanus	2	5		
Protein-energy malnutrition			10	2
Malaria			10	20
Fever/viral		4	2	10
Total deaths	9,164	4,288	4,466	3,298

Note: Columns do not add to 100 because some minor causes of death are not included in the table.
Source: UNICEF 1986.

For Myanmar, which had an infant mortality rate of 49 in 1982, there is good information on the causes of death for infants and children for about the same year (table 3.13). For infants, at least half the deaths occur in the first month of life. Reducing the number of such deaths would require interventions aimed at the mother before and soon after the delivery. Immunizable diseases and parasitic problems do not take a large toll at this early stage. For children age 1–4, acute respiratory infections and intestinal infections (presumably related to parasitic diseases) are the two major problems. Malaria and malnutrition, which are not problems in the first year, begin to take 20 percent of the lives in the older group. For the 5–14 age group, respiratory diseases and malaria are the major problems, accounting for 26 percent of the deaths.

In Myanmar, the following medical interventions have been suggested: higher rates of immunization (which would mainly reduce morbidity, not mortality), more effective basic medical care (to supply better care before and during delivery, to combat acute respiratory infections, and to reduce the effect of intestinal parasites and diarrhea), improved health education for mothers (to improve children's nutrition and better protect them from environmental hazards), better nutrition for mothers and children, improved control of insect vectors to reduce the threat of malaria and parasitic diseases, and safer water and sanitation.[10] From a more general view, these policies revolve around the provision of public health inputs to reduce the incidence of infectious and parasitic diseases, and carefully targeted curative care.

Conclusion

These bits and pieces of information on disease patterns, age structure, differentials in infant mortality by residence and education, and use of health inputs provide little of the detail necessary to set policy within countries, but they do provide a fairly strong base of knowledge for general *directions* for policy. Quite simply, for health sector finance, the principal question is how to target government expenditure to reduce the incidence of communicable diseases, to increase the safety of childbirth, and to increase survival rates among young children. Governments must also find mechanisms to finance the press of curative demands in such a way that they do not prevent the maintenance or expansion of investments in these other areas. The mix of responses may change over time as disease patterns and age structures change, but for most countries in this sample that is not the immediate concern.

There is always the question of whether policy really matters or, put another way, whether a country's financial allocations can make a difference in observed health outcomes. This question is partially empirical, but because we do not yet have strong enough empirical evidence to answer the question, can we provide guidance for health policy on purely deductive grounds? To a limited degree, the answer is yes. First, given the disease patterns discussed here, there is no question that governments are the prime agents of change. Individuals can take measures to protect themselves from malaria or unsanitary environmental conditions, but nothing they can do will be as effective or as economically efficient as community-wide, government activities. Second, some health problems may be difficult to solve without government intervention if they are rooted in misallocations of resources in the home. Given the age and sex groups most at risk—children and their mothers—possible bias against them in the allocation of resources in the home may be a serious problem for some Asian countries. The age and sex mortality patterns shown in figures 3.5, 3.7, and 3.8 differ from the typical patterns elsewhere in the world. These atypical patterns indicate serious underlying resource allocation problems. National goals of reducing population growth, increasing human capital investments, and improving the welfare of women may require that these health problems be solved quickly, and that may require governments to take steps to offset private allocations with targeted subsidies or services. It would be useful to have detailed knowledge of what works in health in different environments and against different disease patterns. In the absence of such knowledge, these general guides to policy can at least point us in the right direction.

We do have examples of precipitous improvements in health conditions. Until World War II, Japan's life expectancy at birth was less than 50 years, approximately where Bangladesh stands today. Today, Japan has nearly the longest life expectancy of any country in the world. China, which was among the poorest and least healthy countries in 1950, made the transition to a level of mortality typical of developed countries in less than 30 years, despite major setbacks along the way. Although increases in income played a role in both countries, there is no question that enormous changes are feasible. Problems of disease are well known, as are the technologies to solve them. In most respects, the speed of success and the character of the interventions come down to a question of policy and how countries choose to spend their health budgets.

Notes

1. In fact, mere availability of such data is a good indicator of effective public health systems and good health conditions. There is some likelihood that the relation is causal in the sense that countries knowing little about disease patterns are unable to take effective steps to alleviate those problems. One author (Hansluwka 1986a) has classified the availability and quality of data for Asia as follows. *Good*: Brunei, China, Hong Kong, Japan, Peninsular Malaysia, Singapore, and Sri Lanka. *Unreliable and/or restricted coverage*: Bangladesh, India, Indonesia, Sabah and Sarawak in Malaysia, Myanmar, Nepal, the Philippines, Republic of Korea, and Thailand. Only 6 percent of the region's population live in countries with reliable mortality statistics, 12 percent live in countries with reasonably good statistics, and another 40 percent live in China (whose recently published statistics for the 1970s and for 1980 are reliable). Thus, nearly half the population of Asia lives where basic epidemiological data are not reliable.

2. One of the major innovations in demography in the 1950s and 1960s was the estimation for developing countries of model life expectancy tables that were based on fragmentary and incomplete data. The cause-of-death tables presented here are from a first effort to create model cause-of-death tables, which are also based on fragmentary data. An important criticism of these tables is that the estimated distribution of deaths by cause is heavily dependent on the epidemiological experience of Europe from 1861 to 1964, which is fairly well documented. Given the major changes in medical technology that have been available to developing countries, their structure of mortality decline may be different from that in Europe, so these model tables should be treated with some caution.

3. These regional classifications are those of the U.N. South Asia is further divided into Middle South Asia and Eastern South Asia. Middle South Asia includes Afghanistan, Bangladesh, Bhutan, India, Iran, Maldives, Nepal, Pakistan, and Sri Lanka. Eastern South Asia includes Brunei, Kampuchea, Myanmar, East Timor, Indonesia, Lao PDR, Malaysia, the Philippines, Singapore, Thailand, and Viet Nam. East Asia comprises China, Japan, Hong Kong, Democratic People's Republic of Korea, Republic of Korea, Macau, and Mongolia. Although these groupings do not conform to the ones used elsewhere in the paper, the data discussed in this section are reported by U.N. region and cannot be reorganized.

4. Obviously there are gray areas that are not covered by these broad statements: (1) many chronic diseases are preventable or can be delayed by public health interventions; (2) the institutional structure required to deliver public health activities may be able to deliver curative services at little additional cost; and (3) the lack of insurance markets for catastrophic events presents an efficiency justification for government intervention in the treatment of chronic diseases. The main point is not destroyed by these qualifications—it is possible to develop a ranking for activities in health that governments should subsidize first. Few people would question that the more "public" aspects of health interventions merit attention first and that these are the types of health problem that characterize high-mortality countries.

5. It has been pointed out to the author that circulatory disease is an odd choice. It is chosen to emphasize the fact that even these chronic conditions are well known to be susceptible to preventive activities, including diet, exercise, and lifestyle. Two recent World Bank health policy documents have emphasized this fact for Brazil (World Bank 1990) and China, countries that have moved swiftly into the low-mortality category. They emphasize that the least-cost role for the government is to emphasize prevention rather than treatment of these chronic problems.

6. Although population projections are available far into the future, and projected age structures up to 2025 and even 2050 have been used in the adult health literature to demonstrate how enormously disease patterns and age structure will change in developing countries over that period, such an approach makes little economic sense. At any reasonable discount rate, the present value of the benefits of investments made, for example, in hospitals to treat patients 20 years in the future will be negligible. Similarly, the capacity of a society to care for larger cohorts of older people in 2025 and later years depends primarily on saving, investment, and technical change—economic growth. On grounds of either health planning or social security, the best strategy may be a certain amount of myopia—that is, investing in solving today's disease problems so that populations are healthier and more productive. Thus the time horizon used in this section—15 years—is relatively short.

7. The United States is included as an example of a country with an older population and low fertility rates.

8. Thailand's numbers in table 3.9 are for five to nine years before the 1975 World Fertility Survey and those in table 3.10 are for up to four years before the survey, which explains the slight difference between the two tables.

9. It is interesting to note that the infant mortality rate in rural areas of Sri Lanka is lower than in its cities, but the probability of dying for children age 1–4 is higher.

10. Other social and economic interventions have been suggested for their potential, if indirect, effects on health, but are not listed here. See UNICEF (1986).

4

Health Care Systems and Patterns of Expenditure

Inputs and outputs in health

In this chapter it quickly becomes clear how important it is to know how good health is produced. If the desired outputs of government health sector activities are certain levels of the World Health Organization's global health indicators, such as life expectancy at birth or infant mortality, the question is what combinations of inputs could achieve those outcomes and how governments in the aggregate are allocating their resources relative to the task.

We know that labor inputs—physicians, nurses, paramedics, and administrators—are needed, but the "correct" proportions are subject to debate in terms of both appropriate technologies and relative input prices. Capital inputs—hospitals, clinics, vehicles, cold chain facilities, and diagnostic equipment—are necessary, but again, the relative quantities required are subject to debate about the appropriate mix from technical and cost standpoints. Specific technologies—such as modern contraceptives, oral rehydration therapy, immunizations, antibiotics, and other more esoteric techniques (kidney dialysis, for example)—are known to have specific effects and entail known costs, but rarely are the implications of these technologies for complementary (and costly) inputs of labor, capital, and supporting infrastructure well understood when health projects are designed.

Almost any goal can be accomplished using different techniques and combinations of inputs. Schistosomiasis, a parasitic disease, could be reduced through the heavy use of labor inputs to change environmental conditions or through less use of labor but greater inputs of chemicals and drugs. Malaria can be attacked environmentally through changes in housing, preventive drug treatment, or hospitalization. All approaches are used simultaneously in practice, but we know little of the relative costs and effectiveness of each approach and the priorities that should be attached to it.

Often we start with a technology (immunizations) or a piece of capital (a rural clinic) and attempt to discover what is necessary to deliver the technology or to staff the clinic according to a desired pattern, assuming that these inputs require additional "ideal" amounts of complementary inputs, such as drugs. These decisions are usually made with little reference to prices or to alternative methods to achieve the same goal. Supporting the technology or the clinic often becomes the goal rather than combating the underlying health problem on a sustainable basis.

Only in a very rough way can we discuss the overall production function for health in the Asian sample. But it is useful to try to identify the outputs that are most needed and the inputs that are likely to make a difference. The previous chapter considered disease patterns in developing country populations, with an attempt to generalize to the Asian sample. It also considered changes in the age structures of Asian populations into the next decade, and examined some issues related to infant and child health. A major conclusion is that infectious and parasitic diseases will continue to be an important concern. Asian health programs that are obviously critical would therefore be activities to prevent and treat these diseases, as well as activities aimed at younger age groups and women of childbearing age, the two groups who bear the brunt of preventable health problems in most of the Asian sample.

This chapter discusses inputs and spending patterns in the Asian sample. Only marginally can we further explore this issue of producing better health with the available inputs, because the necessary numbers are simply not available. The assessment of the cost and impact of health interventions would benefit from rigorous application of benefit-cost analysis or cost-effectiveness analysis, in planning health sector projects as well as household survey work. However, we are not at a complete loss for criteria against which to evaluate spending priorities because the theory of public finance provides a useful framework within which to attach priorities to some government activities in the health sector.

Public health and public finance

The point of departure for evaluating the economic efficiency of government activities in health from a public finance perspective translates almost directly into health professionals' distinction between public health interventions and personal health services oriented to acute health problems. Table 4.1 provides a rough outline of categories that distinguish between the two. The most important aspect of this distinction is that there are a large number of services (category 1)—data collection, health sector planning, health education, health information systems, regulation, and the whole panoply of sanitation, water, and environmental activities—that for the most part are neither exclusive[1] nor rival[2] in consumption and thus are activities that the government must carry out. Many of these activities can have strong redistributive effects because, in the absence of adequate government spending, the poor tend to be

Table 4.1 A public finance approach to government activities in health

Category 1
Public health activities
Epidemiological data collection
Health system planning
Health education
Regulation, licensing
Environmental health
Prevention of communicable diseases
Decreasing cost of utilities (water, sanitation)
Category 2
Mixed public/private activities
Targeted health problems (merit goods[a])
• Family planning
• Maternal/child health
• Infant nutrition
• Immunizations
Treatment of communicable diseases
Category 3
Private activities
Acute care
• Inpatient
• Outpatient
Laboratory services
Hospital hotel services

a. *Merit goods* is an ill-defined concept for labeling goods that society deems desirable, and that the government finances or delivers, notwithstanding the standard economic criteria of efficiency and equity.

least able to compensate for the problems targeted by the spending. Economists have emphasized the importance of these public health activities as a priority for governments in developing countries because the causes of many health problems lie within this sphere.

Category 2 creates major problems for defining reasonable pricing and subsidy activities by governments. When an individual contracts a communicable disease, treating the symptoms has dimensions of a private good, but preventing the spread of the disease is a public health problem. The government has an interest in preventing the disease in the first place, but once it is contracted by someone, both the government and the individual have an interest in curing it—the former to prevent further spread and the latter to get well. Disease prevention through immunizations is a classic example of the dual nature of these activities. Individuals are happy to pay for immunizations, but if immunizations are not subsidized or required by law, people may under-invest in them from a public health standpoint. Communicable diseases that could be controlled might not be because of a failure of individual action. This failure can be eliminated by government action, but it does not mean that the government should "crowd out" all private action.

Category 3 is an area of health in which the private sector can be expected to take primary responsibility. Such services as outpatient care are both exclusive and rival in consumption. If the government becomes involved in the provision of these services, on efficiency grounds it should attempt to emulate the behavior of private firms in charging for the services. Subsidies must be justified with great care. But even here developing country conditions pose special problems that may justify public subsidies to a greater extent than one would predict from a simple application of the theory of public finance. The central economic aspect of any serious acute care problem is that it carries with it substantial risk of large medical bills and loss of earnings. Health financing systems in industrial countries are in fact driven by this fact and the economic complications it creates. In developing countries the lack of structures to make insurance feasible—high administrative costs, low proportion of formal sector employment (with regular paychecks and easily identified, insurable groups)—is the basis for arguments justifying direct government provision or subsidies in some cases, especially in rural areas. But government provision does not mean free provision, and there is no obvious reason for the government to crowd out private provision of the same services.

Finally, as Nancy Birdsall (1989) has pointed out, the institutional structure required to deliver public elements of the first and second groups of activities may be able to provide many of the third group of activities at little additional cost. That is not a reason to provide them for free, but it could reduce the marginal cost enough to make the services relatively inexpensive. The other side of the argument also has merit. Private providers who supply category 3 services could potentially deliver category 1 or 2 services at little additional cost. Thus governments might find it less expensive to subsidize provision of category 1 or 2 services through the private sector than to construct the infrastructure to deliver those services itself.

Under any circumstances, even if we know little about the production function for health, this typology provides a basis for attaching priorities to what the government should do with its money, and it provides guidance for pricing its services. The many health problems that fall into the gray area (category 2) are not exceptions that prove the public/private classification useless. Partial government subsidies may be justified for these activities, but complete elimination of private action makes little sense. The essence of the classification is not the groupings in the table as much as the concepts of rivalry and excludability in consumption on which it is based, and those concepts help in understanding the role of the government in the provision of almost any good—on efficiency grounds, that is.

Some argue that this view of the government role in the health sector is too simple because peculiarities of market structure permeate medical markets. These oddities include the presence of risk, the fact that an agent (the physician) makes many of the treatment decisions for consumers (there is little room for consumer sovereignty), the need for quality control of personnel and drugs, and the fact that health services cannot be traded between individuals once purchased. In any of these areas, government regulation or provision of medical services may be justified, but there is a range of alternatives. A clear black-and-white choice between government and private sector action in the gray areas simply does not exist in practice, and the wide range of institutional arrangements actually used in countries in the sample is testament to this fact. Among the many institutional solutions that have been put in place around the world in response to these market failures in health care, ranging from completely nationalized systems to completely private systems (but always with large government subsidies), none has achieved unmitigated success in offsetting the negative effects. All have introduced new problems, so flexibility in applying the public/private distinction or any other classification system seems warranted, especially for category 2 services.

The attractive aspect of this public health/public finance view is that it shows how improvements in efficiency and, to a lesser extent, equity, can be effected through central policymaking decisions in the health sector—decisions that are for the most part budgetary. And because the disease patterns in most of the Asian sample require category 1 activities, the importance of focusing government action in these areas deserves to be highlighted.

Aggregate resources devoted to health relative to GNP

The data in this section document the aggregate size of government and private spending on health relative to GNP. The numbers are culled from secondary sources that are listed after table A.15 in the appendix.

Health spending in GNP and its composition

Health expenditure in the Asian sample countries varies from 1.4 percent of GNP to 5.1 percent (table 4.2 and figure 4.1), with a regional mean of 3.1 percent. The mean is somewhat less than half of the 7 to 8 percent of GNP spent on health in industrial countries.[3] Korea spends about 5 percent of its GNP on health care, about one percentage point more than does its nearest rival, India. Seven countries—China, India, Korea, Malaysia, Myanmar, Papua New Guinea, and Thailand—all spend more than the group average. These seven are a disparate mix of low-income and middle-income countries, with no particular pattern in either the size or the composition of expenditure. The group that spends the least, which includes the countries with the worst performance in improving health indicators—Bangladesh, Bhutan, and Nepal—spend less than 2 percent of GNP on health care. The remaining three—Sri Lanka, Indonesia, and the Philippines—spend below the mean but more than 2 percent of GNP.

Table 4.2 Aggregate health expenditure and components as a percentage of GNP in selected Asian countries, latest year
(percent)

Country	*Total health expenditure*	*Private health expenditure*	*Government health expenditure*	*Insurance*	*Year*
Bangladesh	1.7	1.0	0.7	0.0	1987
Bhutan	2.0	0.7	1.2	0.0	1986
China	4.0	1.2	0.8	2.0	1987
India	4.3	2.5	1.6	0.2	1987
Indonesia	2.4	1.4	0.9	0.1	1986
Korea	5.1	3.4	0.6	1.1	1987
Malaysia	3.5	0.8	2.7	0.0	1987
Myanmar	3.2	2.0	1.1	0.0	1986
Nepal	1.4	0.5	0.8	0.0	1987
Papua New Guinea	3.8	0.3	3.4	0.0	1987
Philippines	2.4	1.7	0.6	0.1	1987
Sri Lanka	2.3	0.9	1.3	0.0	1986
Thailand	3.8	2.6	1.1	0.0	1987
Mean	3.1	1.5	1.3	0.3	
Median	3.2	1.2	1.1	0.0	

Note: Figures for Malaysia are extrapolated from data for 1983 because no more recent data have been published. Figures for the Philippines are extrapolated from 1985 for the same reason. If the structure of expenditure in those two countries has changed significantly, the picture provided here may be inaccurate for them. For all countries, published figures generally had to be adjusted to increase comparability with the rest of the sample, and private and insurance spending were estimated for some countries. The details are in the relevant appendix tables.
Source: Appendix tables A.9 and A.12.

Public spending accounts for more than half of total spending in 5 of the 13 countries: Bhutan, Malaysia, Nepal, Papua New Guinea, and Sri Lanka. In this group, the public sector accounts for 58 to 91 percent of total spending. For the rest of the sample, where government spending is less than half of all spending, it ranges from a low of about 12 percent in Korea to a high of 40 percent in Bangladesh. The two countries with the lowest direct spending by government, China and Korea, also have the best developed insurance systems.

Although little analytical insight can be gleaned from the distribution of spending across countries, figure 4.1 does raise questions that are important for policy and should be better understood.

• *Public/private mix.* Often the public/private mix of health spending is considered a crucial issue in health. Many evils are attributed to relatively high levels of private spending, including that it results in high total spending, but little commensurate improvement in health, and in the poor distribution of health services. It would not be possible to draw such a strong conclusion for this sample. Papua New Guinea and

Figure 4.1 Health expenditure by source as a percentage of GNP in selected Asian countries, most recent year

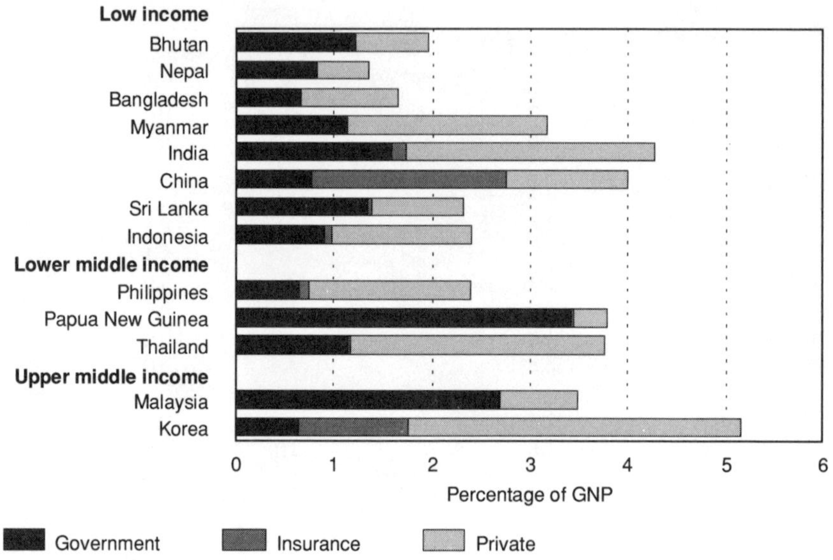

Note: The countries are arranged in order of increasing income per capita, with each group of countries representing about double the GNP per capita of the middle country of the group above it.
Source: Appendix table A.9.

Thailand, for example, spend nearly identical percentages of GNP on health but with a completely different public/private mix. Both countries have improved their health indicators substantially over the past two decades. The other country in that income group, the Philippines, has relatively low spending on health even though a high percentage comes from the private sector.

The importance of the public/private mix may be limited to the simple question of how much the government can and will spend on health. If the government spends relatively little, as in Bangladesh, Nepal, Indonesia, and the Philippines, individuals will compensate by spending relatively more. If the government spends a lot, as in Malaysia and Papua New Guinea, individuals respond by spending less. The variety of experience in the sample appears to cover nearly every possible combination; the broad mix of public and private spending evident in this group does not lend itself to simple dictums about the "correct" proportions.

Two things are certain, however. First, if government spending is relatively high, the government has enormous scope to reduce its share. This is not a normative statement. Whether governments should reduce their share is not an issue—but it is obvious that high spenders crowd out private spending and *could* reduce the size of the bill absorbed by the government.

Second, countries with low public spending coupled with low overall spending risk spending too little on health from government coffers. This statement is more normative, and it relies on the public/private distinctions made in the introduction to this chapter. Because of the limitations of private action in solving environmental health problems and controlling the transmission of communicable diseases, governments must take an active role in order to control infectious and parasitic diseases effectively. If government spending is low, its priorities must be single-mindedly to devote itself to solving these problems first with the available resources. If allocations are inconsistent with this priority, a corrective policy response may involve both an increase in allocations and a reordering of priorities.

An extremely low level of government spending (in this sample, less than 2 percent of GNP) raises warning flags: can spending be increased, and are priorities carefully defined for the inadequate resources currently devoted to health? We do not have a known standard of the minimum necessary level of spending, but we do know that countries devoting less than 2 percent of GNP to government health programs fall into the lower tail of the distribution for Asia.

- *Different spending patterns and similar results.* Sri Lanka and China, often cited for having achieved enviable gains in the health sector, illustrate that different spending patterns can achieve similar results. Sri Lanka is somewhat wealthier, but China devotes a share of GNP to health nearly two times greater than the share of GNP that Sri Lanka spends on health. In Sri Lanka the government is the most important actor in the health sector, and the country has always provided free health services for everyone. In China direct government spending on health (as a percentage of GNP) is among the lowest in the sample. The country has historically recovered costs in government facilities for most curative services. Insurance spending is the highest in the sample.[4]

As was emphasized by the World Bank's first study of the health sector in China (Jamison and others 1984), prevention has been the hallmark of China's government health policy. The small portion of spending channeled through state budgets has emphasized controlling communicable diseases. During the 1980s anti-epidemic stations alone accounted for 15 percent of central government spending on health, according to an internal World Bank report. This number cannot even be extracted from available documents for most other countries in the sample, indicating the relatively low level of attention devoted to this most public of government activities in the health sector. In Indonesia control of communicable diseases accounted for 5 percent of state spending in 1985–86 (according to an internal World Bank report), declining to less than 4 percent two years later. Central government spending on communicable disease programs in India in 1983 was 4.5 percent of health and family welfare spending (see table 6.2 in chapter 6), about a seventh of the amount spent on secondary and tertiary services. About 85 percent of this spending was on malaria control programs alone. States in India spent 12.8 percent of their health and family welfare budgets on communicable disease control, about a fourth of their spending on secondary and tertiary services. We do not know how much should be spent on communicable disease control, but the example of China suggests that this part of a health program can absorb a large share of resources with good results. Analysis of the variability of public health spending and health outcomes across Indian states could provide insights on this question.

• *Private spending and insurance*. Countries with high private spending but little insurance coverage, including Bangladesh, India, Myanmar, the Philippines, and Thailand, could reduce the risks for those incurring large private bills by moving toward the development or expansion of risk-sharing systems. These may include social security systems, encouragement of private insurance, rural cooperative systems, or government-sponsored risk-sharing pools.

There is good reason for concern when countries spend less than 2 percent of their GNP on health; that is far below the mean for the sample. The three countries in that group are by far the worst performers in terms of overall health indicators. And there is some question whether the countries with extremely high spending (in this sample, 4 percent and over), including India, China, and Korea, could reduce it. Are those countries getting their money's worth?

Evidence for China and Korea presented in internal World Bank reports suggests that their spending is headed toward much higher levels with little commensurate improvement in mortality, although this spending may purchase less morbidity and more palliative care. India's high spending is a surprise; its total spending as a percentage of GNP is more than China or Sri Lanka have ever spent on health, but it has failed to achieve results that are remotely comparable.

Countries whose governments spend low levels on health should probably be concerned with the composition of that spending, and governments that spend relatively high amounts can entertain the possibility of reducing the public share. For those countries whose spending falls in the middle, the question of composition and total spending is more complex. But in all cases decisions about changing the composition of spending require detailed analysis of budgets, health sector priorities, and household expenditure patterns beyond what is possible in making these aggregative comparisons. Finally, there is clearly an efficiency gain to be made by introducing risk-sharing schemes in countries with high private spending but little insurance coverage.

Total health spending in dollars

In the previous section, comparability across countries was aided by discussing spending as a percentage of GNP. But that approach does not show the amount of resources devoted to health. For example, India devotes a percentage of GNP to health almost twice as high as does Indonesia, yet Indonesia has almost twice India's GNP per capita. Are both consequently devoting about the same spending per capita to health? In this section, spending is converted to U.S. dollars in order to show how the share of GNP translates into actual resources.

Converting local currencies to dollars using exchange rates creates its own problems. Converting expenditures to dollars tends to underestimate the quantities purchased in developing countries in absolute terms because their prices for untraded goods and services (particularly for labor inputs) tend to be lower than in the United States. The real purchasing power of health expenditures in terms of dollars is consequently understated for all countries in the sample and more so for the poorer ones.

But this distortion does not prevent us from comparing countries. Within the set of low-income countries, dollar amounts should be roughly comparable, as they should be within the set of middle-income countries. Thus less attention in this section should be paid to absolute dollar amounts than to *the position of one country relative to another.*

In absolute dollar amounts, per capita spending for the sample translates into less than 3 percent of health spending in the industrial countries. Even if converting local currencies to dollars understates what these countries get for their money, the large difference between what the sample countries and the industrial countries spend still represents a huge disparity in real resources devoted to health.

Within the sample, the five middle-income countries have 4.5 times the GNP per capita of the low-income countries and spend 5.5 times as much per capita (in dollars) on health. Among the poorer countries, spending per capita ranges from $2 in Nepal to about $13 in India (table 4.3 and figure 4.2). Bangladesh and Nepal are low-level outliers even in that group, spending about a third as much per capita as Myanmar, the next lowest in the group.

The success of China and Sri Lanka in achieving good health outcomes is all the more extraordinary when their spending is compared with that of India (which has about the same level of income) and Indonesia (which is slightly wealthier). Although India and Indonesia spend about the same amount on health per person as China and Sri Lanka, their female life expectancy is still at least 12 years less and their infant mortality more than twice as high as in the other two countries. A comparison of per capita government spending on health—$4.63 in India, $3.90 in Indonesia, $2.13 in China, and $5.40 in Sri Lanka—shows that governments in both India and Indonesia control sufficient resources to achieve ambitious goals. Moreover, government spending in both countries is only 37 percent of total spending on health, which means that government programs can leverage relatively high levels of private spending to achieve goals in the sector. The quantity of resources devoted to health is probably not a major impediment to improving health in India and Indonesia, but how government funds are spent is a pivotal policy issue.

Among middle-income countries, the Philippines, the laggard in improving infant

Table 4.3 Per capita health expenditure in U.S. dollars and share of expenditure by government in selected Asian countries, most recent year

Country	*Health expenditure per capita (U.S. dollars)*	*Government spending as share of all expenditure (percent)*	*Year*
Bangladesh	2.81	40	1987
Bhutan	..	63	1986
China	11.0	19	1987
India	12.5	37	1987
Indonesia	10.4	37	1986
Korea	148.4	12	1987
Malaysia	58.5	77	1987
Myanmar	6.4	36	1986
Nepal	2.1	61	1987
Papua New Guinea	26.2	91	1987
Philippines	14.1	27	1987
Sri Lanka	9.2	58	1986
Thailand	32.8	30	1987
Mean	27.9	45	
Median	11.0	37	

.. Not available.
Source: Appendix table A.12.

mortality in that group, has health expenditure closer to that of the low-income group than to that of the other middle-income countries. It has nearly twice the per capita income of China and India but spends only a few dollars more per capita on health. Government spending, at $3.76 per capita, is a little over a third of Thailand's and less than that of India, Indonesia, and Sri Lanka. The Philippines could spend much more on health, especially from government funds. Government spending is an even smaller portion of total spending than in India and Indonesia; thus, the Philippines has similar opportunities to mobilize private resources in pursuit of health sector goals. But because public spending is relatively low, the major policy question (apart from increasing the level of public support for health) is whether the few resources available are being targeted to public health problems.

Finally, Korea is really in a class by itself in this sample because it has joined the developing Asian economies that are quickly moving to high-income status (Korea is probably more comparable to Hong Kong, Singapore, and Taiwan, China, than to any countries in this sample). In 1982, Korea's GNP per capita was virtually the same as Malaysia's, but a mere five years later it was 50 percent higher (World Bank 1984 and 1989d). Its relatively lavish spending on health is probably a reflection of its income growth, but the question often asked about the United States must also be asked about Korea. Is it getting its money's worth in the health sector, and what steps could be taken to assure that it does?

Figure 4.2 Per capita health expenditure by source in selected Asian countries, most recent year

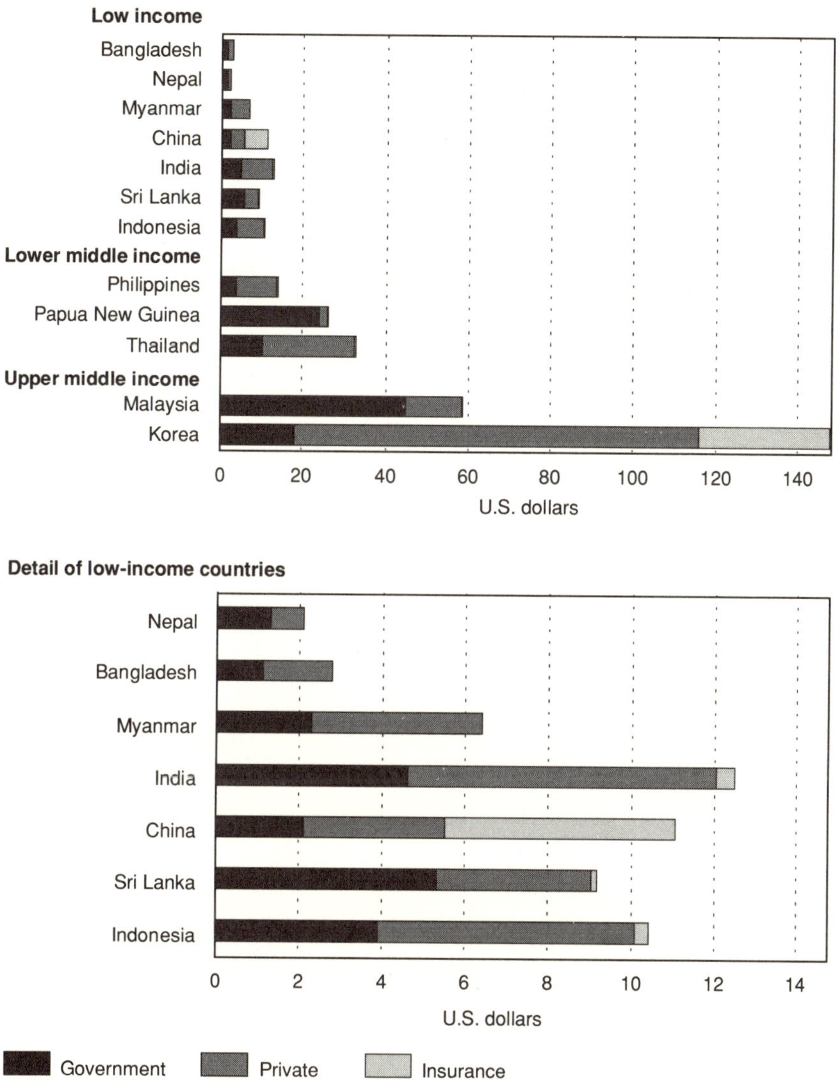

Source: Appendix table A.12.

The relation between total health expenditure and GNP per capita

Underlying the above discussion is a fuzzy idea that, although there is no correct amount of spending for each country at its particular level of income, comparisons can be made among countries that put their spending in perspective. This section adds some rigor to the idea by relating health spending statistically to GNP per capita. We can predict the level of spending for each country given the relation between GNP per capita and health spending that characterizes the entire sample. This prediction is the level of spending that would occur if each country behaved roughly like the average for the sample.

The equation below is estimated using observations for the sample of 12 countries (Bhutan is dropped). The double log specification means that the elasticity of per capita health expenditure with respect to per capita income is given directly as the estimate of α_1 in the equation:

$$\ln (\text{health expenditure per capita}) = \alpha_0 + \alpha_1 \ln (\text{GNP per capita}) + E.$$

Table 4.4 contains results for four estimations, using the above equation but different samples. These are aggregative data, so the high R-squares shown in the table are expected (GNP per capita explains about 90 percent of the variance in health expenditure per capita), and the high t-statistics emphasize the strong relation between health spending and GNP.[5] Figure 4.3 displays these results graphically.

Table 4.4 Regression results for total health expenditure per capita

Regression	α_0	α_1	*t-statistic*	*R-square*	*Sample size*	*Corresponding line in figure 4.3*
Full sample	-5.41	1.31	11.91	0.93	12	Solid
Without Korea	-4.97	1.23	8.79	0.90	11	
Without Korea and Malaysia	-5.54	1.33	7.00	0.86	10	Dashed
Without Bangladesh and Nepal	-4.46	1.17	9.00	0.91	10	Dotted

Source: Author's calculations.

For the full sample, the estimated elasticity of health spending with respect to per capita GNP is 1.31 (a 1 percent increase in GNP is associated with a 1.31 percent increase in health expenditure). If Korea is excluded, the elasticity falls to 1.23. If Malaysia is also excluded, the elasticity rises to 1.33. Although Korea seems to be an outlier, these estimates suggest that Malaysia is also an outlier. Virtually the same predicted line would be drawn whether these two countries are included or excluded, as can be seen by the slight difference between the solid and dashed lines in figure 4.3. In addition, Korea and Malaysia are largely irrelevant to the position of the predicted line at the lower tail of the figure, where the same relation prevails whether they are in or out.[6] The area of most interest is in the lower tail.

Figure 4.3 Relation between per capita income and per capita health expenditure in selected Asian countries
(U.S. dollars)

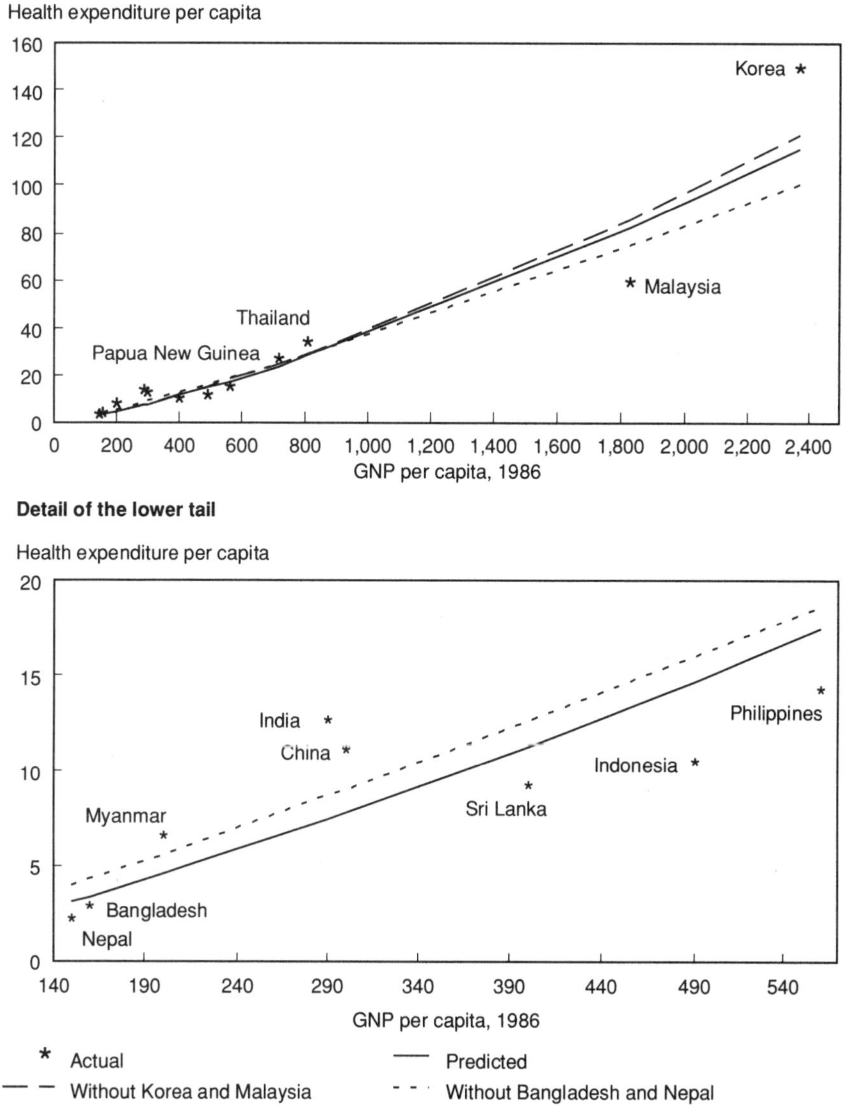

Note: See table 4.4 for key to figure.
Source: Table 4.4.

China, India, Korea, Myanmar, Papua New Guinea, and Thailand spend more on health than would be predicted by per capita income (no matter which line is chosen), and the others spend less. Bangladesh and Nepal are just slightly below the line at the bottom left, but the question arises whether their low spending distorts the predicted line by pulling it toward them. If they are eliminated from the estimation, the predicted line snaps up toward Myanmar in an almost parallel shift at the low end of GNP per capita, which is easily seen in the detail. Because spending is so low at that end of the scale, this small shift corresponds to a large percentage difference in predicted spending. The range in predictions for Nepal is from $3.09 per capita (when Bangladesh and Nepal are included) to $4.01 per capita (when Bangladesh and Nepal are excluded). Actual spending is $2.10. The range may be wide, but even the lowest estimate is 47 percent above current spending.

Table 4.5 shows actual and predicted per capita expenditure for each country using the estimation that excludes Bangladesh and Nepal. Bangladesh, for example, spends $2.81 per capita on health from all sources; if the country were on the dotted line (predicted), it would spend $4.33 per capita. The difference between actual and predicted spending is $1.52 per capita. The last column indicates that Bangladesh would have to spend an additional $161 million on health to bring it up to the prediction for its level of GNP per capita. India, on the other hand, would have to reduce its spending by about $3 billion to move down to the prediction.

Table 4.5 Actual and predicted health spending per capita and gap between them for selected Asian countries, most recent year
(U.S. dollars)

Country	*Actual per capita health expenditure*	*Predicted per capita health expenditure*[a]	*Amount to be added to (+) or cut from (-) actual spending to bring it to predicted spending*
Bangladesh	2.81	4.33	+160,878,633
China	11.00	9.01	-2,125,639,668
India	12.50	8.66	-3,061,560,406
Indonesia	10.40	15.98	+927,736,979
Korea	148.40	100.56	-2,013,917,868
Malaysia	58.50	74.37	+261,776,697
Myanmar	6.40	5.61	-29,890,545
Nepal	2.10	4.01	+33,657,804
Papua New Guinea	26.20	25.03	-4,314,875
Philippines	14.10	18.67	+266,868,973
Sri Lanka	9.20	12.61	+54,837,964
Thailand	32.80	28.72	-218,523,426
Total for countries with shortfall			+1,705,757,051

a. Predicted expenditure was calculated using the estimation that excludes Bangladesh and Nepal.
Source: Author's calculations; see appendix table A.19 for the full set of predictions.

Our concern is only with countries with shortfalls in spending; within that group, however, Sri Lanka and Malaysia, which have done well in the health sector, are not of particular concern. That leaves Nepal, Bangladesh, Indonesia, and the Philippines. For the entire sample, the annual shortfall in spending is $1.7 billion, and these four countries account for 81 percent of that amount. On the plus side, the huge dimensions of "excess" spending in India, Thailand, and Korea indicate that those countries face extraordinary opportunities in the health sector for channeling apparently adequate resources to solving specific health problems.

The relation between government health expenditure and GNP per capita

The next step is to perform the same estimation using government spending rather than total spending as the dependent variable. In this estimation, something had to be done about the distorting effect of insurance expenditure in China and Korea. Insurance was removed from the total by allocating it to government and private spending according to the ratio of those two categories for each country. The operating assumption is that if insurance did not exist, its share of expenditure would be absorbed by the government and private individuals in proportion to their current spending. In addition, the regression was run without China and Korea to test for the effect on the results of their relatively heavy use of insurance as a financing mechanism. As before, Bangladesh and Nepal were also removed to test their effect on the estimates. Results for three estimations are shown in table 4.6 and illustrated in figure 4.4.

Table 4.6 Regression results for government health expenditure per capita

Regression	α_0	α_1	*t-statistic*	*R-square*	*Sample size*	*Corresponding line in figure 4.4*
Full sample	-5.63	1.20	7.50	0.85	12	Solid
Without Korea and China	-6.72	1.39	7.32	0.87	10	Dashed
Without Bangladesh and Nepal	-4.86	1.09	5.19	0.77	10	Dotted

Source: Author's calculations.

Per capita GNP explains government health spending exceedingly well. Both the R-square and t-statistic are close to the high levels that characterized the estimates for total spending in the previous section. When the entire sample is used, the elasticity of government spending with respect to GNP per capita is 1.2, slightly lower than for overall spending. When Korea and China are removed, the elasticity rises to 1.39. When Bangladesh and Nepal are removed, it falls to 1.09. These two results are almost mirror images of one another—low government spending at the upper tail tends to pull the predicted line down; low government spending at the lower tail

Figure 4.4 Relation between per capita income and per capita government health expenditure in selected Asian countries
(U.S. dollars)

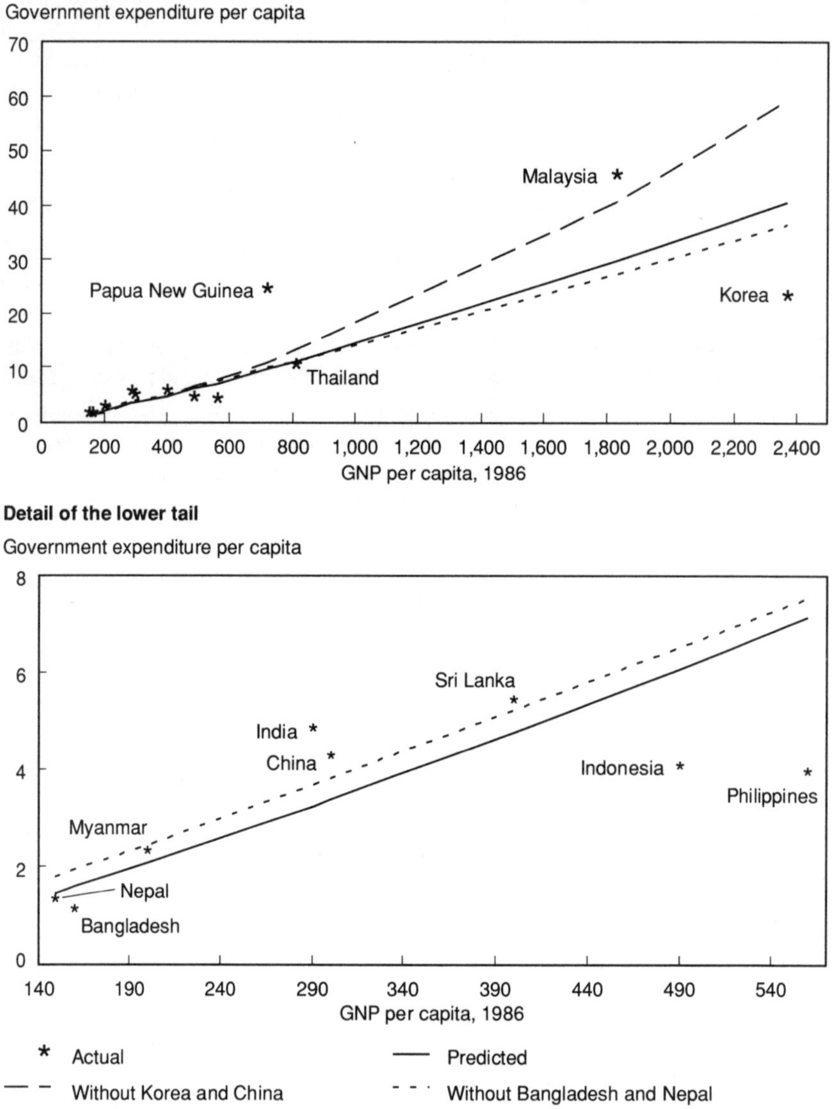

Note: See table 4.6 for key to figure.
Source: Table 4.6.

tends to rotate the estimated line upward. We are more concerned with low spending at the bottom of the tail, so the line without Bangladesh and Nepal will be used in the subsequent discussion.

Table 4.7 shows the difference between actual and predicted government spending. This is the part of spending the government can do something about directly. The same four countries cited as having shortfalls in total spending—Bangladesh, Indonesia, Nepal, and the Philippines—also have shortfalls in government spending relative to what would be predicted for them. Three other countries—Korea, Myanmar, and Thailand—have shortfalls that are more than compensated for by surplus private spending (the difference between total spending and government spending). Malaysia and Sri Lanka, which both have a shortfall in total spending, have surpluses in government spending that do not completely offset their lower-than-expected private spending (suggesting that for them a dollar of public spending crowds out more than a dollar of private spending, which may be considered good, bad, or irrelevant).

The total annual shortfall in government spending is nearly $800 million, and 91 percent of this amount is accounted for by the four countries that have deficits in both government spending and total spending. Pushing Nepal and Bangladesh up to their predicted levels of government spending would cost about $95 million annually and would remove half the deficit in total spending. The annual cost of pushing Indonesia's government spending up to the trend is much higher, nearly $500 million annually. It would cost about $200 million to push the Philippines' spending up to the predicted level.

Figure 4.5 shows the distribution of the shortfall between the public and private sectors for these four countries. The depth of the problems in the public sector in the

Table 4.7 Actual and predicted government health spending per capita and gap between them for selected Asian countries
(U.S. dollars)

Country	*Actual per capita health expenditure by government*	*Predicted per capita health expenditure by government*[a]	*Amount to be added to (+) or cut from (-) government health budget to reach predicted level*	*Percentage of total shortfall*
Bangladesh	1.12	1.93	+86,003,203	10.8
China	4.24	3.82	-446,006,720	
India	4.81	3.68	-897,727,749	
Indonesia	4.02	6.51	+415,141,508	52.2
Korea	22.91	36.12	+556,326,433	
Malaysia	45.00	27.28	-292,458,869	
Myanmar	2.29	2.46	+6,474,069	0.8
Nepal	1.28	1.80	+9,148,947	1.2
Papua New Guinea	23.79	9.90	-51,401,916	
Philippines	3.92	7.53	+210,953,796	26.6
Sri Lanka	5.40	5.23	-2,809,596	
Thailand	10.00	11.25	+66,949,939	8.4
Total shortfall			794,671,462	100.0

a. Predicted expenditure was calculated using the estimation that excludes Bangladesh and Nepal.
Source: Author's calculations; see appendix table A.20 for the full set of predictions.

Philippines is striking. The government accounts for about 80 percent of the shortfall in spending. In Bangladesh the government's share is about half, and in the other two countries it is much smaller.

Although these estimates are discussed in terms of shortfalls or surpluses, they should not be taken as standards against which to judge spending levels. The intention has been to give a quantitative picture of where countries stand relative to each other. Almost nothing has been said about those that spend more than is predicted for them; the overriding concern is with those whose spending is low, and with how much it would cost to increase their spending. There is also no reason to stop when the increments to spending discussed here are achieved. By increasing spending, the countries below the predicted line will cause the line to move up, more than likely leaving them below it even then. Predicted spending is thus a moving target. Furthermore, continually increasing spending may be unnecessary inasmuch as the goal is improved health, not higher spending. To have Sri Lanka's or Malaysia's health indicators and fall below the predicted level of spending, as both countries do, is certainly not a situation requiring correction.

Health expenditure by different levels of government

Figure 4.6 disaggregates government spending into expenditures by central governments and local or provincial governments as a percentage of GNP. Papua New Guinea stands out as a country in which large government expenditures appear to be largely local in origin; in fact, almost all funding to local governments for health is earmarked and provided by the central government. Increasingly, however, provincial governments are raising supplementary funds for health services. In China and

Figure 4.5 Government and private sector shares in the shortfall in health spending in selected Asian countries

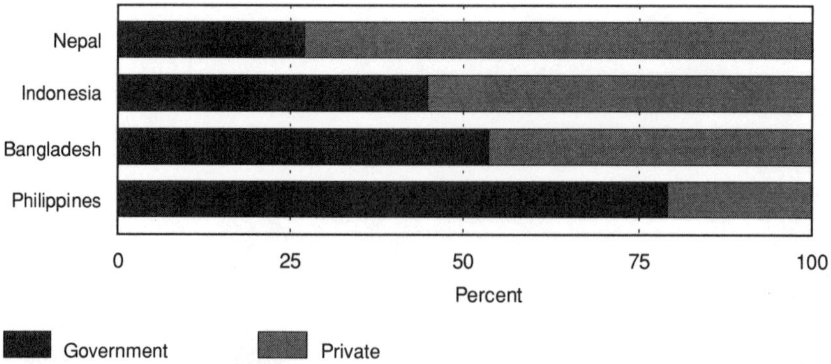

Source: Appendix tables A.19 and A.20.

Figure 4.6 Health expenditure by level of government as a percentage of GNP in selected Asian countries, most recent year

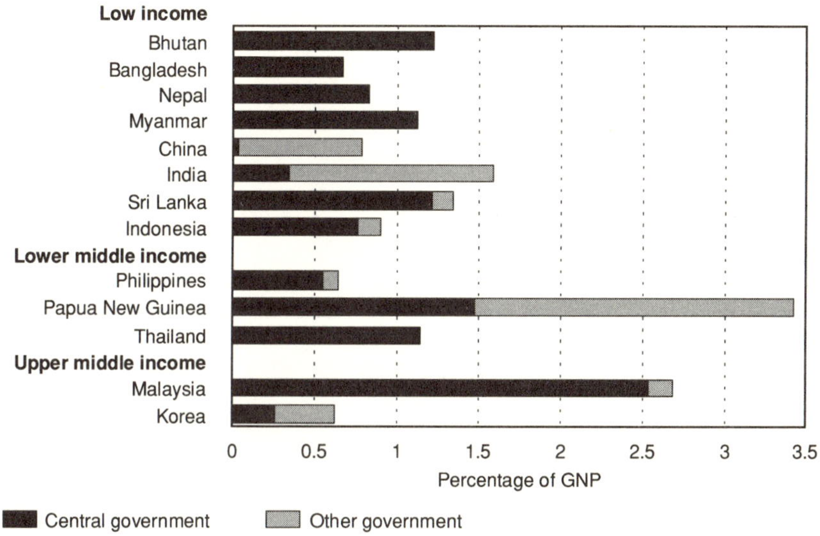

Source: Appendix table A.9.

Korea—countries with relatively low public spending on health—central government spending makes up less than half of all public spending. India stands out as another country in which the central government controls considerably less than half of public spending in the health sector. These three countries use very pluralistic financing systems for health. The countries with the worst health problems and the lowest spending on health services appear to have no little or no local capacity to raise money for health care.[7]

Trends in government spending

Table 4.8 shows trends in government spending as a percentage of GNP. In real terms, all governments are spending more on health in total. Even a constant share of GNP over time in each country corresponds to higher spending in real terms because real GNPs have been rising. Whether the increase in total resources is enough to offset population growth is another question.

Only 5 of the 12 countries increased the percentage of GNP devoted to government health programs consistently over the 12-year period covered in table 4.8, despite greatly increased concern with health and population programs. Among those, only Papua New Guinea and Thailand have significantly increased spending as a percentage of GNP. Most of the countries are spending approximately the same

Table 4.8 Government spending on health as a percentage of GNP in selected Asian countries, 1975, 1980, and latest year

Country	*1975*	*1980*	*Latest year*
Bangladesh	0.5	0.8	0.7
China	0.7	0.9	0.8
India	1.6	1.2	1.6
Indonesia	0.2	0.7	0.9
Korea	0.4	0.5	0.6
Malaysia	2.6	2.4	2.7
Myanmar	0.8	0.9	1.1
Nepal	0.7	0.6	0.8
Papua New Guinea	2.6	3.2	3.4
Philippines	0.6	0.5	0.6
Sri Lanka	1.6	1.5	1.3
Thailand	0.5	0.9	1.1

Source: Appendix table A.8.

proportion of GNP on government health programs that they spent in the mid-1970s. Sri Lanka has cut its spending as a percentage of GNP continuously over the period, but it still ranks fourth from the top. Allocations in countries that have performed below the mean for the sample in reducing infant mortality, which include Bangladesh, Indonesia, Nepal, and the Philippines, are also the only countries in the sample (other than Korea) that have consistently spent less than one percent of GNP on government health activities.

Figures 4.7 and 4.8 show government spending for the low-income and middle-income countries in nominal U.S. dollars over the 11 to 12 years covered by the data. The scale of the two figures is radically different, and the countries are shown in order of increasing per capita income. The governments of India, Korea, Myanmar, Papua New Guinea, and Thailand have increased spending per capita, in nominal U.S. dollars, consistently since 1975; whether the increases are enough to offset inflation is a question that cannot be answered here because it requires that the analysis be carried out in the local currency. Only China has decreased nominal government spending per capita during the 1980s. Although spending in Bangladesh, Indonesia,[8] and the Philippines has been stable, in real terms per capita spending by the governments in these countries must have, at best, stagnated. These are three of the four governments identified in the previous section as falling well below the spending levels that would be predicted for them on the basis of per capita income. Sri Lanka cut spending between 1975 and 1980, but it has recovered since then (at least nominally).

Composition of government spending

The share of total government spending going to health ranges from a low of 2.2 percent in Korea to 10 percent in Papua New Guinea, with a regional average of 5.2

Figure 4.7 Government health spending per capita in selected low-income Asian countries, for selected years, 1975 to most recent year

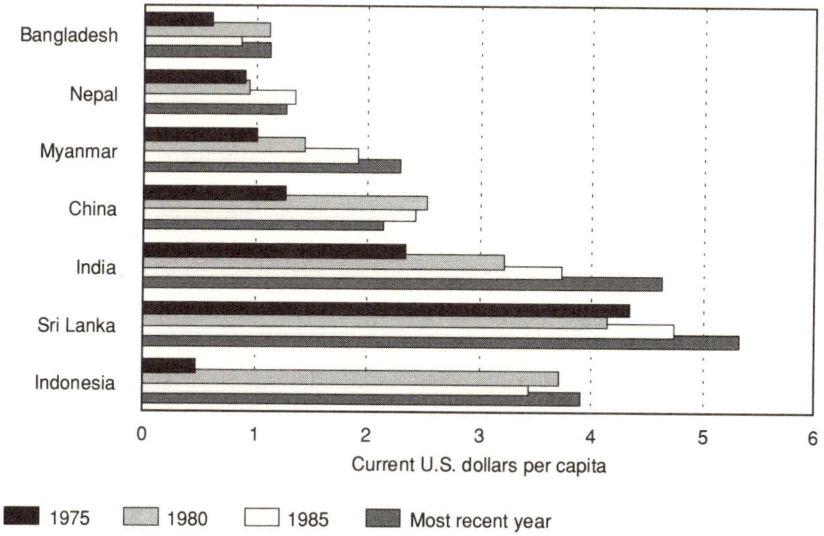

Source: Appendix table A.12.

Figure 4.8 Government health spending per capita in selected middle-income Asian countries, for selected years, 1975 to most recent year

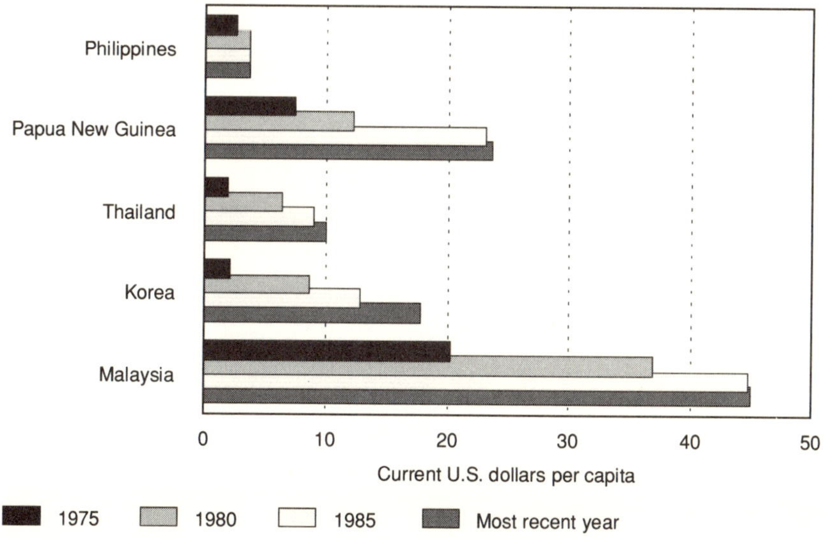

Source: Appendix table A.12.

percent. Apart from Korea, the governments of Bangladesh, Indonesia, and the Philippines make the smallest efforts in health relative to the budget. Malaysia spends heavily on health from government coffers: 6.8 percent of all spending by the government goes to health. India, Myanmar, and Thailand nearly match this effort, which is something of a surprise.

The allocations of spending between hospitals and other programs reported in table 4.9 are somewhat dependent on the accounting practices of health ministries and on how subsidies for other programs supporting the health system (such as medical education) are distributed across government departments. For example, if only direct spending on rural, district, and national hospitals in Bangladesh is included in the total, the allocation to secondary and tertiary facilities reported in the table (56 percent) is correct. If spending on medical and nursing schools, as well as on administration and supplies, is allocated to the hospital system, well over 80 percent of the health budget would be attributed either directly or indirectly to hospitals. As another example, Papua New Guinea has mandated that less than half of government health allocations will be spent on hospitals; although this rule has resulted in difficult spending decisions, it has also been accommodated by the relabeling of some facilities (previously called hospitals) as health centers. Using a

Table 4.9 Government spending on health in selected Asian countries, most recent year
(percent)

Country	Health spending as share of total government spending	Share in health budget, by type of facility		Share in health budget, by type of expense		
		Secondary and tertiary hospitals	Clinics, primary and public health	Salaries	Nonsalary expenses	Capital expenses
Bangladesh	3.9	56	44	51	23	26
China	4.2	67	33	18	56	26
India	6.7	71	29	51	42	7
Indonesia	3.8	59	41	39	36	25
Korea	2.2	50	50	8	57	35
Malaysia	6.8	59	41	67	19	14
Myanmar	6.8	33	67	29	36	35
Nepal	4.3	50	50	53	37	10
Papua New Guinea	10.0	43	57	68	28	4
Philippines	3.3	58	42	43	51	6
Sri Lanka	4.5	70	30	44	44	12
Thailand	6.1	58	42	48	29	23
Mean	5.2	56	44	43	38	19
Median	4.4	58	42	43	37	19

Source: Appendix tables A.10 and A.14.

conventional definition of a hospital would increase the allocation attributed to them substantially. Another type of problem is posed by Korea. An important component of its central government spending on health is its support of the medical aid system, which provides health subsidies to assist in paying medical bills for the indigent. That spending accounts for most of the share listed under hospitals (it also explains why salaries are such a small portion of expenses). Because public hospitals in Korea recover their costs from patients, these costs are for the most part not counted under government expenditure. Thus Korea's numbers are really not comparable with those from the other countries.

Given these qualifications, some of the patterns are as expected. Well over half of government spending, on average, goes to hospitals. China and Sri Lanka, both low-mortality countries, spend heavily on hospitals, well above the average for the sample. Malaysia, which also has achieved good health indicators, spends a much smaller proportion of its budget on hospitals, but the difference may be attributable to the youth of its population relative to that of China and Sri Lanka (see figure 3.10) and to the fact that the data for Malaysia are based on the distribution of expenditure in 1983. A major surprise is that despite relatively high mortality, India's spending pattern, with 71 percent of government spending absorbed by hospitals, is similar to patterns in these low-mortality countries.

Other than Papua New Guinea, only Myanmar spends less than half its government budget on hospitals. Most of the others spend close to the mean of 58 percent. There are at least two ways to interpret this phenomenon. One is that some minimal institutional structure of hospitals, physicians, and nurses is a fixed cost of a public health system. Countries such as Bangladesh and Nepal, where total government spending is low, may devote high proportions of government budgets to hospital care because of these high fixed costs, over which they may have little control. If hospitals are a fixed cost, the issue of a relatively high proportion of the budget being spent on them is one of total budgets being too small. In fact, there is little evidence to support this idea. If hospitals were a fixed cost of a health system, expenditure on them would rise as a percentage of the budget as budgets fall. Although Myanmar spends only a dollar more per capita than Bangladesh and Nepal, however, only a third of its budget goes to hospitals. India spends four times as much as Bangladesh and Nepal, but 71 percent of its budget goes to hospitals.

A second, more plausible interpretation is that the share going to hospitals is a variable that reflects a choice and that countries currently spending a high proportion of their budgets on hospitals (despite poor performance on health indicators) have made inappropriate allocation decisions. The variability of the figures even for this small sample is consistent with the idea that a large share of hospital spending is a matter of choice. In the Philippines, for example, about half the hospital beds are in the private sector, and insurance covers about a third of hospital expenses (for half the population). Yet the government spends 58 percent of *its* health budget on hospitals, much of which must be redundant. India also has a large private sector, many intransigent public health problems that are firmly locked into category 1 of table 4.1, and a serious female mortality problem. Yet it spends public funds on hospitals as if life expectancy were 20 years longer than it is.

Capital budgets at this level of aggregation are dominated by new construction; maintenance is relatively inexpensive. Bangladesh, China, Indonesia, Korea, and Myanmar appear to be spending heavily to expand their systems. Several countries—India, Papua New Guinea, and the Philippines—have such low capital spending that maintenance of the existing physical plant must be in even greater jeopardy than is typically the case.

The general implication of table 4.9 is that governments are allocating large shares of their spending to category 3—acute care—services. There is a high likelihood that, from a public finance perspective, this is an inefficient allocation of public resources, more so for countries with lower spending and worse health outcomes.

Institutional context and issues in hospital economics

Institutional features

All countries in the sample have government health systems that consist of hospitals, clinics, field-workers, and public health programs. These exist side by side with private fee-for-service allopathic and traditional sectors that provide medical care, drugs, and midwifery services. There are also charitable and mission facilities that operate for the most part outside the government's system, although they sometimes receive subsidies.

Statistics on the size and scope of activities outside the government sector that could be compared across countries are generally unavailable, as are data on clinics, field-workers, and vertical programs in the government sector. We do, however, have fairly standardized information on the number of hospitals and hospital beds in both the public and private sectors for the sample, although the quality of the data varies considerably and provides an imprecise picture of the current situation. This section focuses on the available hospital statistics. Hospitals account for 50 percent or more of government health care spending in most of the countries, so at least we are able to provide some detail on the most important component of spending.

Hospital economics

In the Asian sample, an average of 79 percent of the hospital beds are in the public sector, and there are almost 1,400 people per bed (table 4.10). The population-to-bed ratios, except for those in Bangladesh and Nepal, compare well with those in other developing regions.[9] The distinctions made between public and private are fragile. In China, for example, although 100 percent of the beds are in the government sector,

Table 4.10 Public and private hospital beds in selected Asian countries, most recent year

Country	*Total hospital beds*	*Population per bed*	*Government hospital beds as percentage of total*	*Beds per hospital*		
				Govern-ment	*Private*	*Govern-ment multiple*
Bangladesh	29,566	3,589	85	63	..	..
China	2,296,819	465	100	35	..	..
India	535,735	1,489	74	96	42	2.3
Indonesia	95,450	1,743	69	154	117	1.3
Korea	75,388	558	18	94	167	0.6
Malaysia	37,939	435	86	322	28	11.6
Myanmar	25,599	1,484	100	41	..	..
Nepal	3,902	4,511	86	42	51	0.8
Papua New Guinea	4,793	772	100	251	15	16.8
Philippines	90,279	647	53	78	35	2.3
Sri Lanka	43,759	368	91	83	..	..
Thailand	80,620	665	90	109	23	4.8
Mean	1,394	79	114	60	5.1	
Median	719	86	89	39	2.3	

.. Not available.
Source: Appendix table A.15.

most hospitals are administratively autonomous units that attempt to recover costs, in many cases fully.

The number of beds per hospital gives an idea of the distribution of public hospitals in the country—if the average number is low, government hospitals are likely to be dispersed. That is because governments tend to add to hospitals in cities rather than to build new facilities in the same area. Although private hospitals are small, they are not necessarily more dispersed because they gravitate to cities and are often extremely small facilities owned by one or two private doctors. The median size of government hospitals for the whole sample—89 beds—is fairly small, given the fact that virtually every country contains a few giant hospitals with several thousand beds. Indonesia, Malaysia, and Papua New Guinea appear to be exceptions to this statement, with fairly large public hospitals on average. But the difference may be due more to different definitions of hospitals in those countries than to significant differences in this pattern of small, dispersed government hospitals. Hospitals in Bangladesh, China, Myanmar, and Nepal are on average extremely small, with 60 or fewer beds.

Studies of hospital costs in developed countries have generally concluded that there are increasing returns to scale for small hospitals (those with fewer than 100 beds, certainly for any with 50 or fewer beds) and constant or slightly decreasing returns to larger hospitals. Very large hospitals (with thousands of beds and comprehensive services) appear to face decreasing returns to size (in terms of beds). In other words, costs per patient day on inpatient wards tend to fall as hospitals with few beds become larger, but beyond about 100 beds there is little or no effect of size on costs until hospitals become very large. At some point, they become uneconomically large. This is an oversimplification, but it does convey the flavor of the relation between hospital size and costs in developed countries.[10] There are other cost issues that should capture our interest, such as the following:

- Do costs fall as occupancy rates go up for a given size of hospital?
- What are the tradeoffs between hospital size and occupancy rates, or when is it more economical to build a new hospital rather than to expand an old one?
- Do costs for different services fall as some are combined in the same facility?

There are no general answers to any of these questions because so few studies have been done of hospital costs in developing countries (Barnum and Kutzin 1990 count five statistical cost studies: China, Ethiopia, Kenya, Nigeria, and Peru). Yet even these few studies provide some guidance. First, very small hospitals (certainly those with fewer than 50 beds) are probably more costly places to treat inpatients than are larger facilities. Second, costs per patient can fall as occupancy rates rise if occupancy is low to start with. When new personnel and supplies are required to treat additional patients, however, costs will begin to rise. Third, hospitals can become too large, and costs could probably be cut by building new facilities rather than adding more beds or departments to gigantic facilities. Fourth, there is little disaggregated evidence on the economies of having different specific departments within the same hospital. Some analysis of the effect of inpatient services on the cost of outpatient care is enlightening, however. Hospitals seem to increase the cost of outpatient services by using more expensive inputs. That the more expensive inputs have a significant effect on results for the typical patient is unlikely.

For the most part, these suggestions merely provide hypotheses that should be tested in each country, and the resulting information should be incorporated into hospital planning. Directions for policy that are most important for this sample of countries are the following:

- On average, the size of government hospitals in this sample falls well within the small category, which implies that about half the government hospitals are quite small from an economic standpoint. There may be opportunities to reduce hospital costs by consolidating some small rural hospitals. Governments would be sacrificing the broader distribution of hospitals for lower patient costs, but they would in the process increase the potential quality and variety of services available in a smaller number of facilities. In Asia, where population densities are high and transportation facilities have improved enormously in the past decade, more centralized rural facilities may make more sense than in other parts of the world.
- The single gigantic national hospital that is typical in small countries (and in a

number of cities in the larger countries) is probably uneconomically large. Such hospitals could be profitably reduced in size, and some of the services they provide could be distributed more broadly in the country. Plans to expand these large hospitals, which are common, should be carefully examined.

- It is probably not economically efficient to expand hospital outpatient departments in either urban or rural areas; in fact, for most outpatients a hospital setting is not required, and it probably raises treatment costs.

Just how important each of these concerns may be for this sample will become clearer below, when spending per government hospital bed is estimated. The results from economic studies, however tentative they may be, are notable because they tend to contradict typical government policies with respect to hospitals—wide dispersion of small inpatient facilities, concentration of high-level inpatient care in a small number of giant facilities, and concentration of urban outpatient care in local hospitals.

Government hospitals in Asia tend to be much larger than private hospitals (table 4.10). The size of government hospitals as a multiple of the size of private hospitals can be interpreted as a rough indicator of the development of the private sector. If government hospitals are substantially larger than private hospitals, it is probable that the most sophisticated hospitals are in the public sector and that private hospitals are small primary care operations. In countries in which the government accounts for virtually all hospital beds, the multiple is infinite, and it tends to fall as the private sector accounts for a larger part of the total. The range in the subsample in which some private facilities exist is from 0.06 in Korea and 0.08 in Nepal, two countries where public hospitals are on average smaller than private hospitals, to 11.6 in Malaysia and 16.8 in Papua New Guinea, two countries where the private sector is virtually undeveloped. In countries where this number is high, there is wide scope for private sector involvement, which is one method for reducing the burden of hospitals on government budgets.

Government hospital expenditure

Table 4.11 contains information on expenditure per *government* hospital bed and patient day. These estimates are calculated from the aggregate spending statistics presented in the section in this chapter on the aggregate resources devoted to health relative to GNP. They are not the result of cost-accounting exercises in the hospitals.

The procedure for creating these numbers is simple. We know how many dollars the government spends on health and the fraction going to hospitals. Multiplying those numbers and dividing by the number of government hospital beds yields the average expenditure per bed, the first column of numbers. Dividing that number by per capita income yields the multiple of per capita income per bed in the next column. Similar calculations, taking into account overall occupancy rates, yield

Table 4.11 Expenditure on government hospital beds and patient days in selected Asian countries, most recent year
(estimated)

Country	*Expenditure per bed (U.S. dollars)*	*Multiple of annual per capita income per bed*	*Bed occupancy rate*	*Expenditure per day occupied (U.S. dollars)*	*Percentage of annual per capita income per day*
Bangladesh	2,661	17	67	10.88	6.8
China	665	2	91	2.00	0.7
India	6,650	23	80	22.77	7.9
Indonesia	5,822	12	55	29.00	5.9
Korea	27,881	12	60	127.31	5.4
Malaysia	13,474	7	63	58.59	3.2
Myanmar	1,122	6	97	3.17	1.6
Nepal	3,371	22	70	13.19	8.8
Papua New Guinea	7,886	11	68	31.77	4.4
Philippines	2,658	5	77	9.46	1.7
Sri Lanka	1,508	4	84	4.92	1.2
Thailand	4,270	5	80	14.62	1.8
Mean	6,497	10	74	27.31	4.1
Median	3,820	9	74	13.91	3.8

Source: Appendix table A.15.

estimates of the cost per day per occupied bed and the percentage of yearly per capita income required to pay for each occupied government bed every day (the last two columns in the table).[11]

The average cost per bed is quite high ($6,497), but that is heavily weighted by Korea's and Malaysia's high spending.[12] Myanmar and Sri Lanka spend relatively little per bed. China's exceptionally low figure probably reflects the low budgetary cost of hospitals that are largely self-supporting. It makes sense to use the median for comparison because of this distortion in the distribution. Costs in Bangladesh, Nepal, and the Philippines are at least 50 percent higher than in China, Myanmar, and Sri Lanka, but less than the median. India, Indonesia, Papua New Guinea, and Thailand are well above the median.

When the expenditure is divided by per capita income, a more useful metric appears. On average, countries in the sample spend 10 times their per capita income to support each government hospital bed every year. The range is from 2 (China) to 23 (India).

Figure 4.9 displays this statistic relative to the sample median of 9 times per capita income. The center of the graph (at 0) is the median, so each bar shows the deviation from the median. Bangladesh, for example, spends 17 times its per capita income on each bed, 8 multiples more than the sample median. The length of its bar is therefore 8, not 17. Sri Lanka spends 4 times its per capita income per bed, or 5

Figure 4.9 Multiple of per capita income spent on government hospital beds for selected Asian countries, relative to the sample median

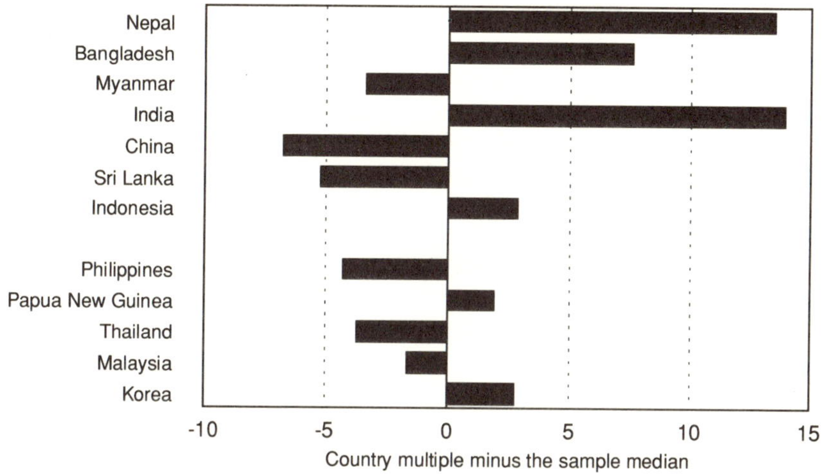

Source: Author's calculations.

multiples less than the sample median. Its bar has a length of –5. The ordering of countries is by per capita income.

The low-income group contains the countries spending both the most and the least per bed. Bangladesh, India, and Nepal spend far more than the sample median. For Bangladesh and Nepal, this outcome is due not so much to high spending per bed as to low per capita income. For India, it is due to some of both. China and Sri Lanka, it will be recalled, devote relatively large shares of their budgets to hospitals; this graph suggests that they get a lot of services for their money. The richer countries, in contrast, spend large absolute amounts on hospitals, which turn out to be a small multiple of per capita income. They spend a lot more than the poorer countries but they can also better afford it.

Figure 4.10 incorporates the bed occupancy rate into the calculations. Countries with relatively low occupancy rates perform relatively worse on this measure, but the ordering is essentially unchanged from figure 4.9. Indonesia's low occupancy rate pushes its costs higher; China's and Sri Lanka's high occupancy rates push their costs farther below the median.

Government hospital expenditure and disease patterns

This picture of costs is not complete without incorporating some idea of how hospitals are used. An illustrative analysis is performed in this section for Myanmar. Not only is the necessary information available only for Myanmar, it is also a good

Figure 4.10 Percentage of per capita income spent on occupied government hospital beds per day for selected Asian countries, relative to the sample median

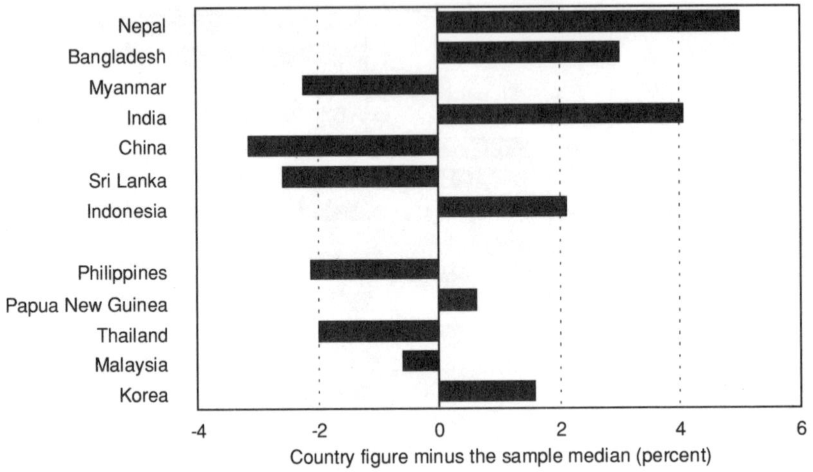

Source: Author's calculations.

choice because it allocates the smallest fraction of the government budget to hospitals in this sample, it has high bed occupancy rates, its beds are relatively inexpensive in terms of local resources, it ranks at about the middle of the group in life expectancy and infant mortality, and its improvement in those indicators has been relatively fast over the last two decades. In short, Myanmar's hospitals command relatively few resources, they are relatively cheap and efficiently used, and the country has done well in improving health conditions.

Table 4.12 shows total patient days for nine disease categories in 435 out of 619 public hospitals in Myanmar in 1981. Patient days are multiplied by Myanmar's daily cost of an occupied bed in 1986 ($3.17) to get the total cost of inpatient hospital services for each illness category. The diseases appear in descending order according to total cost. These nine disease categories account for 57 percent of all cases; the other 43 percent enter under the undefined "other causes" category, for which costs could not be calculated because the average length of stay was not available for that group.

Several general observations should be noted. First, none of the expensive chronic disease problems characteristic of industrial country hospitalizations—circulatory diseases and cancers—even appears as a separate category on this list. They cannot represent more than the 43 percent of cases lost in the "other causes" category. Second, nearly all the conditions in the table are preventable or are the object of other health sector interventions. These include malaria; tuberculosis; abortion;[13] about two-thirds of the admissions for digestive ailments; and a sizable fraction of the accidents, ill-defined fevers, respiratory infections, and skin infections. Third, although the government spends on average $2.29 per capita, it is easy to see that this spending is captured for the most part by individuals when it is channeled into curative services. Each tuberculosis case, for example, at $81 per episode, requires 35 times the government's spending per capita to treat. As a result, roughly 0.04 percent of the population being treated in hospitals for tuberculosis absorbs 1.4 percent of the government's health budget. Without doubt those who absorb this spending and those who pay for it would be better off if the expenditure became unnecessary. Fourth, this table includes only direct treatment costs. Each of these illnesses imposes additional costs on the individual and society in forgone wages, reduced pleasures of life, and increased risks for families. These indirect costs are likely to dwarf direct treatment costs.

The last three columns of the table show spending by disease relative to total spending for this group, relative to total hospital spending, and relative to the total health budget. Because the patient day statistics come from only 70 percent of government hospitals, the last two columns are lower-bound estimates. Hospital-based malaria treatment alone accounts for more than a fifth of all expenditure for

Table 4.12 Inpatient spending in government hospitals, by condition, in Myanmar

Condition	*Total patient days*	*Total cost (U.S. dollars)*	*Cost per case (U.S. dollars)*	*Spending as percentage of total for this group of conditions*	*Spending as percentage of total government hospital spending*	*Spending as percentage of total government health spending*
Malaria	697,883	2,211,575	20	23.4	7.7	2.5
Digestive	496,425	1,573,161	19	16.6	5.5	1.8
Obstetrical	412,842	1,308,287	15	13.8	4.6	1.5
Respiratory	399,951	1,267,435	24	13.4	4.4	1.5
Tuberculosis	373,138	1,182,467	81	12.5	4.1	1.4
Accidents/injuries	252,157	799,079	19	8.5	2.8	0.9
Fever	217,026	687,752	21	7.3	2.4	0.8
Skin infections	132,174	418,855	30	4.4	1.5	0.5
Total	2,981,595	9,448,612	22	100.0	32.9	10.9
For reference:						
Government cost per patient day				$3.17		
Total hospital spending				$28,722,078		
Government health spending per capita				$2.29		
Total government health spending				$87,020,000		
Hospital spending as percentage of total				33.0		

Note: Disease statistics are for 1981 and are from 435 out of 619 hospitals. Budgetary data are for the most recent year.

Source: Burma, Department of Health 1987, and calculations in this report; see appendix table A.18.

Table 4.13 Population per health professional in selected Asian countries, 1981 and mid-1980s

Country	*Population per physician 1981*	*Population per physician mid-1980s*	*Percentage change*	*Population per nurse 1981*	*Population per nurse mid-1980s*	*Percentage change*	*Population per nurse and midwife mid-1980s*	*Population per assistant mid-1980s*
Bangladesh	9,690	6,731	-31	19,370	18,180	-6	8,984	10,059
China	1,730	1,122	-35	1,670	1,369	-18	1,369	583
India	3,700	2,574	-30	4,670	4,478	-4	1,782	66,796
Indonesia	12,330	9,714	-21	2,300	8,783	282	1,319	3,004
Korea	1,390	1,151	-17	350	580	66	580	20,528
Malaysia	3,910	2,887	-26	1,390	979	-30	979	5,311
Myanmar	4,930	3,683	-25	4,920	4,892	-1	2,255	10,480
Nepal	28,780	33,254	16	33,390	29,940	-10	9,682	9,553
Papua New Guinea	15,610	13,052	-16	930	891	-4	891	11,664
Philippines	6,850	6,730	-2	2,640	2,753	4	2,753	6,848
Sri Lanka	7,460	8,274	11	1,260	1,957	55	1,396	16,549
Thailand	6,870	6,416	-7	2,140	957	-55	826	6,060
Mean	8,604	7,966	-15	6,253	6,313	23	2,735	13,953
Median	6,860	6,573	-19	2,220	2,355	-4	1,383	9,806

Note: The data for population per physician for China include both western and Chinese doctors, while the data for other countries are limited to physicians trained in western medicine, so the absolute numbers are not strictly comparable. But percentage changes across countries should be somewhat comparable even if the positions included in each category are not exactly the same.

Source: World Health Organization 1988 and World Bank data.

this group of diseases and at least 2.5 percent of the entire health budget. It has not been possible to find out how much the government spends on the control of malaria, but it would be surprising if it devotes as much to prevention as to the inpatient costs caused by the parasite.[14] Spending on malaria treatment on an inpatient basis means spending at least 2.5 percent of the health budget to treat 0.29 percent of the population (assuming each case involves a different individual). In contrast, the benefits of malaria *control* are distributed widely across the population.

Conservatively speaking, at least half the hospital expenditure accounted for in table 4.12, nearly 6 percent of the government's health spending, could be avoided if other health sector strategies were successful in reducing the incidence of the infectious and parasitic diseases in this list. (Unfortunately, there is no information on the relative cost of preventive approaches.) If this is the case in Myanmar, with low spending on relatively cheap hospitals and relatively good health status indicators, what is the situation in the high-cost, high-mortality countries? It is extraordinarily difficult to justify spending on hospitals in high-mortality countries, especially when the hospitals are relatively expensive in terms of local resources.

Broad patterns of resource allocation among inputs

Health outcomes are affected not only by aggregate spending levels, but also by the allocation of spending among inputs. Data are generally too patchy, however, to document the distribution of resources except in broad terms. The evidence presented in this section relates to the choice of alternative mixes of labor inputs in producing health services.[15] Although labor is only one among many health inputs, it absorbs a significant share of resources—one that varies highly among countries (as the allocation of public spending in table 4.9 demonstrates).

Trends

Since the early to mid-1980s, population per physician has declined by about a third in Bangladesh, China, and India, with smaller but still substantial declines in Indonesia, Malaysia, Myanmar, and Papua New Guinea (table 4.13).[16] Only in Nepal and Sri Lanka has the supply of physicians relative to population worsened. In Nepal, that is particularly troublesome because the country started the 1980s with the lowest availability of physicians, and its situation worsened both absolutely and relative to its neighbors by the mid-1980s. The Philippines showed little increase in its supply of physicians, but this must be because the reported numbers refer only to government physicians. There is no reliable count of private physicians in the Philippines, but my extrapolation based on a physician survey in the early 1970s indicates that there are at least twice as many doctors as reported, and the supply is probably growing faster than the population.

The figures for nurses in table 4.13 are much less reliable, and to some degree the indicated improvements may be statistical errors. The estimates for population per nurse attempt to match definitions of nurses between the two periods as carefully as possible. Clearly there has been a failure in matching data for Indonesia,[17] and possibly for Korea, but results in the other countries appear to be sensible. Only in Malaysia, Nepal, and Thailand has the quantity of nurses grown faster than the quantity of physicians; elsewhere, the growth in nursing personnel has lagged behind the growth in the more expensive physicians.

If this table is compared with appendix tables showing the figures for 1965, the success of several countries in expanding the supply of personnel in the 1980s becomes even more impressive. Bangladesh and India, for example, actually had a greater improvement in coverage by physicians between 1981 and 1985 than between 1965 and 1981.

Countries that have particularly small supplies of physicians and nurses, especially Bangladesh and Nepal, have substituted midwives (or other workers at that level) and health assistants for doctors and nurses (see the last two columns of table 4.13).

Cross-country differences in labor input mixes

Among indicators of labor input ratios, the ratio of population per health professional, which combines all health professionals, is a reasonably good global index of the overall availability of health services.[18] Bangladesh and Nepal have by far the highest ratio of population per health professional (table 4.14), which corroborates earlier evidence on the underfinancing of health services in these countries. The remaining countries fall into two broad groups: India, Indonesia, Myanmar, and Sri Lanka have moderately high ratios, while the remaining countries have distinctly lower ratios. The Philippines probably also belongs in the latter group since the data presented in the table exclude private sector health personnel, who are estimated to make up about half the total number of practitioners in that country.

Broadly, one can distinguish between several levels of health personnel, ranging from physicians, who generally offer the most sophisticated services, to health assistants at the lower end. From an economic perspective, perhaps the most relevant considerations are that these personnel are generally paid different wages and their training varies in costliness. Thus, the choice of different mixes of health personnel is important in the efficient use of resources.

Consider as a first cut the distribution between more qualified personnel (physicians and nurses) and less qualified ones (midwives and health assistants) (table 4.14, third column from the right).[19] Most Asian countries show a ratio close to unity, the outliers being Indonesia (5.0) and Nepal (3.3). Although these comparisons are highly aggregated and ignore wage differences, they do suggest a possible undersupply of more qualified staff relative to other staff in these two countries.

Table 4.14 Indices of labor input mixes in selected Asian countries, mid-1980s

Country	*Ratio to physicians*			*Ratio of midwives and health assistants to physicians and nurses*	*Ratio of other health personnel to physicians*	*Population per health professional*
	Nurses	*Midwives*	*Health assistants*			
Bangladesh	0.4	0.7	0.7	1.0	1.8	2,414
China	0.8	0.8	1.9	1.5	3.6	246
India	0.6	1.4	0.0	0.9	2.1	842
Indonesia	1.1	7.4	3.2	5.0	11.7	765
Korea	2.0	2.0	0.1	0.7	4.0	229
Malaysia	2.9	2.9	0.5	0.9	6.4	338
Myanmar	0.8	1.6	0.4	1.1	2.7	985
Nepal	1.1	3.4	3.5	3.3	8.0	3,684
Papua New Guinea	14.6	14.6	1.1	1.0	30.4	415
Philippines	2.4	2.4	1.0	1.0	5.9	979
Sri Lanka	4.2	5.9	0.5	1.2	10.7	710
Thailand	6.7	7.8	1.1	1.1	15.5	388
Mean	1.3	2.9	0.6	1.5	4.7	1,386
Median	1.6	2.7	1.1	1.1	6.2	738

Source: Author's calculations, based on table 4.13.

The distribution of physicians relative to all other health personnel in the system shows wider variation (table 4.14, second column from the right). Papua New Guinea is an extreme outlier, with a ratio exceeding 30, suggesting a striking shortage of physicians (or extremely high investment in lower-level staff that is far beyond the point of diminishing returns). This is corroborated by the ratios of physicians to nurses and to midwives. In four other countries—Indonesia, Sri Lanka, Thailand, and, to a lesser extent, Nepal—physicians are also scarce relative to other health workers. The breakdown into the various categories of workers suggests a substitution of nurses and midwives for physicians.

Bangladesh deserves separate comment. The ratio of physicians to other health workers, at 1.8, is the lowest in the Asia region, and is consistent with a health delivery system with a relatively heavy emphasis on secondary rather than primary health care. It is also consistent with a wage structure in which the differences between the most qualified and the least qualified are compressed. In addition, contrary to expectations, the direct cost of training a paramedic in this country is apparently almost as high as training a physician. Under these circumstances, the pattern of personnel input mix is not surprising. However, given the striking deviation from other countries, it does raise questions about the efficient use of health personnel. It is especially interesting to contrast Bangladesh's position with that of Nepal. Both countries show an overall scarcity of health workers relative to other

Table 4.15 International Comparison Project: Relative quantities of medical services consumed in selected countries, 1975 and 1980

	United States	*Japan*	*India*	*Indonesia*	*Korea*	*Malaysia*	*Philippines*	*Sri Lanka*	*Thailand*
Quantity per capita, 1975									
Medical care	100	84	4	..	12	12	10	7	9
GDP	100	68	7	..	21	22	13	9	13
Quantity per capita, 1980									
Medical care	100	112	4	2	15	..	19	14	..
Drugs/appliances	100	62	6	1	41	..	6	29	..
Health services	100	119	3	3	1	..	28	7	..
GDP	100	74	5	9	20	..	17	12	..

.. Not available.

Note: Medical care refers to the entire category. Its components are drugs/appliances and health services.

Source: Kravis, Heston, and Summers 1982 and United Nations 1987.

Asian countries, but in Bangladesh the need is relatively greater for less qualified paramedics than for physicians, while in Nepal the imbalance between physicians and other health workers is less acute.

Price-adjusted comparison of spending on health

Comparisons of health expenditures and their allocation are sensitive to differences in price structures across countries because medical care is labor-intensive and it is not an internationally traded service. In an earlier section in this chapter, these differences were controlled by expressing aggregate spending relative to the GNP; when the discussion turned to exchange rate–converted U.S. dollars per capita, this issue was ignored. In this section, a refinement is added to the discussion by using data from the International Comparison Project (ICP) in which actual price differences have been explicitly taken into account. Although the evidence is fragmentary and somewhat dated, it nevertheless yields insights regarding differences among countries in the quantities of health services consumed, prices, and consumption patterns.

Table 4.15 displays data on relative quantities and table 4.16, data on relative prices, for 1970 and 1980 for Asian countries included in the ICP. For reference, data are shown for the United States and Japan. For ease of comparison, the data for the United States are taken as the numeraire for each of the indicators displayed.[20] Although not all Asian countries in this study are represented in these tables, the International Comparison Project treats those that are included as representative of the price and quantity structures of countries that are near each other geographically and in terms of per capita income. By that criterion, the table is fairly representative of the Asia region. South Asia, Southeast Asia, and East Asia are represented, but China is excluded.[21]

Per capita quantities of medical services produced and consumed

Perhaps the most important lesson from table 4.15 is that comparisons between industrial countries and developing countries significantly understate the amount of medical services actually produced and consumed in the latter. India's total per capita spending on medical services (including both private and government spending) in 1975 was about $4.30 based on the exchange rate—0.54 percent of U.S. spending per capita that year (about $800). If price differences between the two countries are taken into account, as is done in table 4.15, India's per capita spending actually purchased about 4 percent of the quantity of medical services bought in the United States. Four percent is low, but it is eight times higher than the exchange rate–converted dollar amounts would suggest. Koreans spent $32 per capita in 1975, about 4 percent of U.S. per capita spending that year. The quantity purchased, according to table 4.15, was about 12 percent of that in the United States, three times higher than implied by the exchange rate conversion.

Table 4.16 International Comparison Project: Relative prices of medical services in selected countries, 1975 and 1980

	United States	*Japan*	*India*	*Indonesia*	*Korea*	*Malaysia*	*Philippines*	*Sri Lanka*	*Thailand*
Prices relative to U.S. prices, 1975									
Medical care	1	1	0.1	..	0.2	0.3	0.1	0.1	0.3
GDP	1	0.9	0.3	..	0.5	0.5	0.4	0.3	0.5
Prices relative to U.S. prices, 1980									
Medical care	1	0.5	0.1	0.4	0.2	..	0.2	0.1	..
Drugs/appliances	1	0.6	0.5	2.3	0.6	..	1	0.1	..
Health services	1	0.5	0.1	0.2	0.1	..	0.1	0.1	..
GDP	1	1.1	0.4	0.4	0.6	..	0.4	0.2	..
Prices relative to U.S. prices, 1975									
Drugs	1	0.8	0.3	..	0.3	0.7	0.5	0.1	0.4
Medical supplies	1	1.2	0.5	..	0.5	0.6	0.7	0.7	0.6
Therapeutic equipment	1	0.8	0.1	..	0.2	0.2	0.2	0.1	0.3
Physicians' services	1	0.7	..	..	0.1	0.6	0.1	0.1	0.4
Dentists' services	1	0.4	..	..	0.1	0.6	..	..	0.7
Nurses' services	1	0.8	0.2	..	0.1	0.1	0.2	0.1	0.3
Hospital services	1	..	..	..	0.6	0.1	0.1	..	..
Hospital construction	1	1.1	0.2	..	0.6	0.4	0.4	0.2	0.3

.. Not available.

Note: Medical care refers to the entire category. Its components are drugs/appliances and health services

Source: Kravis, Heston, and Summers 1982 and United Nations 1987.

Obviously a direct comparison can also be made across developing countries. The exchange rate–converted numbers cited in the previous paragraph indicate that India consumed about 13 percent as much health care as Korea (4.3/32), but the ICP numbers indicate that it consumed 33 percent (4/12) as much, 2.5 times more. Malaysia and Korea had almost identical consumption patterns in 1975, as did the Philippines and Thailand. Sri Lanka, with its excellent health statistics, was among the lowest consumers of medical services.

This general pattern of smaller quantities of medical services (but not nearly as small as indicated by exchange rate–converted spending) consumed in developing countries also holds for 1980, the latest year for which the comparisons are available. There are some realignments among the developing countries, however. Between 1975 and 1980, the Philippines and Sri Lanka approximately doubled the quantity of medical services consumed per capita relative to that consumed in the United States (consumption also grew in the United States). Korea's consumption rose only slightly, and India's stayed at about the same level. India consumed 57 percent of the quantity of medical services consumed in Sri Lanka in 1975; by 1980 India consumed only 29 percent as much. Generally, consumption of medical goods and services rose faster relative to consumption in the United States than relative to GDP.[22]

Consumption patterns

The numbers for 1980 allow comparison across countries in the distribution of purchases of drugs and appliances (this category will be referred to as pharmaceuticals) and of health services, the two components of medical care in table 4.15. The distribution of consumption between the two categories varies greatly. Filipinos, for example, purchased four times the quantity of health services that Sri Lankans purchased in 1980, but they bought only about a fifth as many pharmaceuticals. Indians purchased about the same quantity of health services as Indonesians, but they consumed six times more pharmaceuticals. Indonesia's consumption of pharmaceuticals was only one percent of U.S. consumption, and Korea's consumption of health services was, surprisingly, only one percent of that in the United States. In contrast, Koreans consumed 41 percent as many pharmaceuticals as Americans. The ratios of drugs and appliances to health services range from 0.21 in the Philippines to 41.0 in Korea, implying large differences in the composition of demand for medical services.

Relative prices

Why would consumption patterns vary so much across countries? Differences are due partly to culture, beliefs, education, and the state of technology. It is also likely that relative prices have a strong effect on the observed patterns. Relative price levels for the same countries, using the same format, are shown in table 4.16.

The difference in consumption patterns between the Philippines and Sri Lanka is

Figure 4.11 Relative prices and quantities of pharmaceuticals and medical services in selected Asian countries, 1980

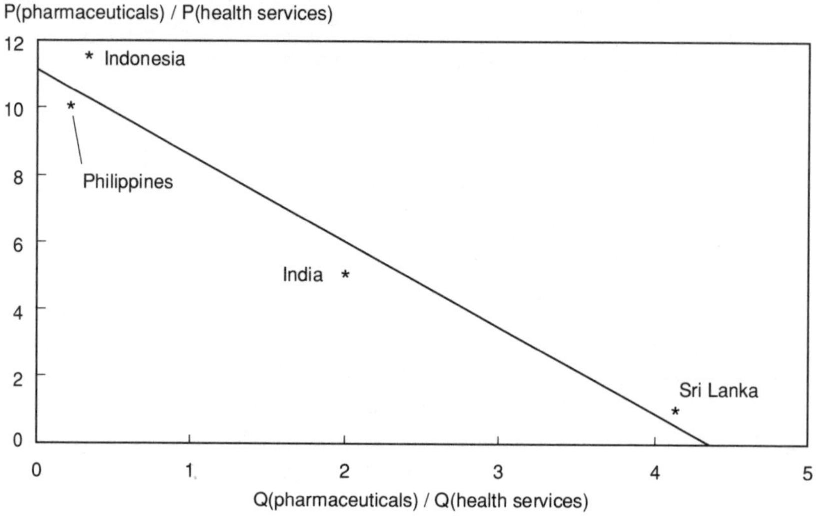

Source: Author's calculations based on tables 4.15 and 4.16.

clearly related to prices. Health services in the Philippines in 1980 cost the same as in Sri Lanka (0.1 percent of the U.S. price in both), but pharmaceuticals were about 10 times more expensive in the Philippines than in Sri Lanka (1.0 percent of the U.S. price in the Philippines and 0.1 percent in Sri Lanka). If the price of pharmaceuticals relative to the price of health services in the United States is taken as 1:1, the ratio in Indonesia was 11:1 in 1980. In other words, pharmaceuticals in Indonesia were 11 times more expensive than health services when compared with the price differential in the United States. No wonder Indonesians substituted health services for drugs! In India, drugs were five times more expensive relative to health services than in the United States. The greater detail[23] provided for 1975 prices in the last section of the table suggests that, relative to the U.S. price structure, drugs and medical supplies were by far the most expensive components of medical care in each of the Asian countries. Only in Korea did some of the other components compete with these.[24]

Figure 4.11 shows the relation between these price and quantity ratios for the sample of Asian countries, excluding Korea.[25] As the price of pharmaceuticals rises relative to the price of health services, there is substitution of health services for pharmaceuticals. The methods chosen to combat illness in these countries appear to be quite sensitive to relative prices.

Overall, the price of health services in 1980 in the developing countries of Asia was 10 to 20 percent of the U.S. price, but the price of pharmaceuticals and therapeutic supplies was 50 to 230 percent of the U.S. price. The range of drug prices excludes prices in Sri Lanka, where they were 10 percent of U.S. prices. One of the main reasons that prices of pharmaceuticals and therapeutic devices are so much higher is that most are traded on world markets and thus reflect more closely international price levels than does the untraded labor used to deliver health services.

Even pharmaceuticals that are produced locally contain imported ingredients that reflect world prices and that are usually taxed at the border. Labor services are largely untaxed in most developing countries. In India, for example, Ahmad and Stern (1987) found that there was no direct government tax on "medical health" but that the effective tax rate was really 21 percent, due exclusively to indirect taxation of inputs used to produce drugs domestically. Out of 80 commodity groups, they found that "medical health" had the fourth highest indirect tax rate in India.

The quantities consumed do not always reflect what might be expected on the basis of relative prices. Koreans, as mentioned in note 25, are heavy consumers of drugs despite their relatively high price. Indians also consume higher relative quantities of pharmaceuticals than might be expected, given the price structure that they face. However, there may be a minimum quantity of drugs that must be consumed to make purchases of health services effective. Because India uses such a low level of inputs, its drug purchases may represent a lower (but expensive) technical bound. If this speculation is true, India's high effective tax rate on medical health is a burdensome tax indeed on the sick.[26]

The high cost of hospital beds in the high-mortality countries that spend low levels on health and these countries' high spending on hospitals is a stunning finding. High-mortality countries that spend half or more of their government budgets on hospitals are diverting at least half of their meager resources to purchase what is for all practical purposes a luxury good (as indicated by the high price in terms of local resources) that benefits only a small share of their populations.

Relative prices are rarely taken into account in designing health programs or in evaluating the performance of those programs once deployed. For example, recent health interventions have in most cases been designed to supply inexpensive technologies—such as immunizations, oral rehydration therapy, and simple drug treatments—in rural areas. These technologies appear inexpensive within the prevailing price structures of industrial countries, where the required drugs and transport services are inexpensive relative to other medical inputs. Yet those inputs may be expensive in poorer countries, especially in the poorest Asian countries.[27]

In Bangladesh, for example, the cost of traditional healers, who usually require no traded inputs (such as modern medicines or syringes), may substantially undercut almost any service connected to allopathic medicine. A 1987 household survey found that rural Bangladeshi households paid on average 0.4 taka for outpatient visits at government clinics; private physician visits cost 6.8 taka, private paramedic visits 2.6 taka, and visits to homeopaths 1.1 taka (Griffin 1989). The government clinic was the least expensive. When drug costs were added, however, the average government visit cost 24.0 taka. With drugs included, private physician visits cost 64.7 taka, private paramedic visits 31.6 taka, and homeopath visits 15.1 taka. Table 4.17 shows these expenditures relative to expenditures at the government clinic, with and without drugs. Not only did the cost of drugs reverse the cost advantage of the government clinic over homeopaths, it also reduced the government's competitive advantage relative to private paramedics and physicians. The basic reason is that labor services are such a small component of expenditures even in the private sector. The government is able to subsidize the cost of the cheap input—labor—but it is less successful in cutting the cost of the expensive input—drugs.

Table 4.17 Cost ratios for various sources of care, with and without drugs, in Bangladesh, 1987

	Costs relative to costs for a visit at the government clinic	
Source of care	*Without drugs*	*With drugs*
Government clinic	1.0	1.0
Private physician	17.0	2.7
Private paramedic	6.5	1.3
Homeopath	2.8	0.6

Source: Griffin 1989.

When health programs in developing countries are evaluated, they are typically faulted for failing to provide adequate inputs of drugs and medical supplies, for budgeting inadequately for maintenance of equipment and vehicles, and for supplying insufficient fuel and parts for transportation and communications. In fact, correcting these shortcomings (as donors often encourage programs to do) may represent a poor budgeting decision given the relative prices of the inputs. In some cases, adequately maintaining vehicles might cost the equivalent of the salaries of several essential employees.

When programs are compared in terms of local prices, medical interventions may turn out to be costly relative to labor-intensive environmental interventions. For example, in rural Bangladesh a Union Health and Family Welfare Center requires approximately $2,000 a year in salary expenses for four workers and is currently allocated approximately $900 worth of drugs (converted at exchange rates). A recent experiment has shown that if an additional $800 is spent on drugs, utilization will increase from current low levels to "desired" levels. The additional $800 is not much money in U.S. terms, but it represents a high resource cost in the sense that the additional expenditure on medicines would approximately equal expenditure on two paramedics.[28] Another way of thinking of it is that each person in the unit must be accompanied by an equal value of drugs to make the clinic operate according to plans. But these are just the direct costs. Additional drugs require other expenditure, on storage facilities, transportation, administration, and security. On the other hand, a hospital bed in Bangladesh costs about the same as one of these clinics (table 4.11).

In contrast, the possible cost advantage of labor-intensive public health programs that use few traded inputs—such as programs designed to promote health education, destroy the habitat of disease vectors, and clean up the environment—may be substantial when the local costs of alternative programs are taken into account. The use of monumental, labor-intensive environmental activities as a health intervention in a country such as Bangladesh (possibly mimicking China's successful effort to control the four pests—rats, flies, mosquitos, and bedbugs—and to control schistosomiasis and malaria) has never been fully explored. Moreover, the often observed failure of local people to change their medical care consumption patterns after government programs are put into place may have at least as much to do with the relative prices they face as with the cultural factors that are commonly cited.

Although many of these statements are speculative, they are designed to provide examples of how important local prices are in:

- Comparing expenditure across countries and understanding what the differences actually mean
- Designing sustainable health programs
- Understanding differences in client and supplier behavior across countries.

Health programs designed according to industrial country technology, staffing standards, or perceptions of quality will be difficult to sustain in the Asian sample because price structures for medical services are so different. More problematic is that programs appropriate to one developing country may not translate easily to other developing countries. Given the different price structures in India and Sri Lanka, for example, a program designed according to relative prices in Sri Lanka, where drugs are relatively inexpensive, would be substantially more expensive in terms of real resources in India, where drugs are relatively costly but labor is inexpensive.

Summary

The preceding discussion draws out significant differences among countries in the region. The role of private sector provision varies widely: although most hospital facilities are government-owned in Asian countries, the breakdown ranges from 100 percent in China, Myanmar, and Papua New Guinea, to only 18 percent in Korea. In terms of health financing, the aggregate resources from public and private sources vary from a low of only 1.4 percent of GNP in Nepal and 1.7 in Bangladesh, to more than 5 percent in Korea. In these three countries, government spending is relatively low, less than 0.8 percent of GNP. In Korea, however, an enormous amount of resources is generated from private sources, placing it ahead of all the other Asian countries in aggregate spending on health. In Bangladesh and Nepal weak administrative infrastructure and poverty may make it difficult to mobilize private resources to the same extent. Thus, while continued efforts would be needed to maintain and expand current levels of private financing, increased government spending also appears warranted in these countries. On the other hand, in Malaysia and Papua New Guinea the aggregate resources for health are moderately high, but the share of government resources in the total is much larger than in other countries in the region (especially in Papua New Guinea), suggesting that public financing may have crowded out private contributions.

With regard to the allocation of resources among health inputs, the data are patchy. Labor costs absorb a large proportion of health spending, so the mix of labor inputs provides a useful insight in this regard. In Bangladesh and Nepal the very high population-to-health worker ratios reflect the paucity of financial resources. But if health personnel are separated into the various categories—physicians, nurses, midwives, and health assistants—an unusually high concentration of physicians relative to other health workers in Bangladesh becomes apparent. Thus, while more health personnel appear warranted in both countries, the expansion in Bangladesh should avoid exacerbating the current imbalance; correcting it would of course be even better, although administrative and political obstacles may stand in the way.

In Bangladesh high expenditure on personnel has contributed to low expenditure on supplies and equipment, which has the perverse impact of making the expensive personnel less effective. In Papua New Guinea, although the government has substituted away from more expensive personnel, it has employed relatively large numbers of workers and maintained employment at a high level by allowing the physical plant to deteriorate. The best performing countries in the sample, including China, Korea, and Sri Lanka, spend well above the mean on nonsalary inputs. Only Malaysia does not fit this pattern among the better performing countries.

The analysis also points to a possible shortfall of better qualified staff in Indonesia, Sri Lanka, Thailand, and, especially, Papua New Guinea. It is ironic that Papua New Guinea spends so much on government health services, yet the private sector in that country is the fastest growing part of the health sector. Physicians are leaving the public service because of low pay, and patients are leaving because of perceived poor quality of care. The reaction of the government has been to explore the possibility of retraining some of the health assistants to become junior physicians, essentially a continuation of the current policy (John Snow, Inc. 1990). Without more information on wage structures, however, it is not possible to confirm that current patterns of personnel use in specific countries are inconsistent with wage structures.

That wage and price differences are responsible for some of the observed variation in health inputs is supported by data from the International Comparison Project. Although somewhat old, the data carry an important note of caution against ignoring price differences when evaluating health strategies. In particular, health interventions and technologies designed for industrial countries cannot automatically be transferred to developing countries because of vast differences in price structures for health inputs. Even among developing countries, these differences remain large, pointing to the need to adapt strategies to local conditions.

Notes

1. In essence, excludability means that the good or service can be physically held back from someone who does not pay for it. A pharmacist may refuse to provide aspirin to a customer unless payment is made first. Aspirin is exclusive in consumption. However, if person A pays for mosquito control, person B cannot be excluded from the benefit even if he or she pays nothing. Thus, mosquito control is not exclusive in consumption. Person B has an incentive to "free ride" on person A.

2. A good or service is rival in consumption if the benefits flowing to the person purchasing it are reduced if others also try to receive some of the benefits. In health, if person A pays for and consumes aspirin, the benefits of that aspirin are not available to person B. If person B attempts to gain benefits from the aspirin, it can only be accomplished by reducing the benefits flowing to person A. Aspirin is a rival good. However, if person A pays for mosquito control, person B can benefit from it without reducing the benefits flowing to person A. Mosquito control is not rival in consumption. In fact, because it is both nonrival and nonexclusive in consumption, it fails the private market test on both grounds and qualifies as a pure public good. The result is a failure of individual action—collective or government intervention is required.

3. Seven to eight percent is the average if countries are taken as the unit of analysis. When weighted by population, the figure for industrial countries is approximately 11 percent of GNP.

4. Much of the modern sector of China's economy is owned by the government, and health insurance is mandated for most of those enterprises, so some might argue that what is called insurance there is essentially government financing of curative services for the modern sector. Nevertheless, the payment mechanism is through insurance, not through direct government spending. The institution paying for the care (the insurance system) is different from the institution providing the care (government hospitals). In the past, the government focused its financial involvement in curative care on assisting enterprises and rural communities to develop risk-sharing arrangements, in subsidizing hospital care for indigents, and subsidizing rural doctors (almost exactly the prescription a neoclassical economist would give for central government activities). In the early 1980s, in a country that would probably be considered too poor to have insurance at all, only 30 percent of the population was completely uninsured. Thus, there is little question that the government succeeded in its efforts to pay for the bulk of inpatient care through the insurance mechanism.

5. The high t-statistic implies that the relation observed is extremely unlikely to be a spurious statistical phenomenon.

6. Analysts using larger samples of countries, including industrial countries, have produced similar estimates of the elasticity of health spending with respect to GNP. Schieber (1987) regressed per capita health spending in OECD countries against GDP per capita in 1984 and found that a 1 percent increase in GDP per capita predicted a 1.4 percent increase in per capita health spending (his numbers were in purchasing power parity equivalents rather than the exchange rate conversions used in this paper). Schieber's results are roughly comparable to results obtained from a larger sample of countries for the mid-1970s under the International Comparison Project (Kravis, Heston, and Summers 1982). ICP estimates of price and income elasticities for medical care across countries were -0.5 and 1.4, respectively. The negative price elasticity means that across the sample of countries, a 1 percent increase in the price of medical care causes an 0.5 percent drop in medical care purchases. Asia's spending pattern relative to income is broadly consistent with these other estimates for the world as a whole, including the richer countries.

7. This point is relevant inasmuch as primary health programs attempt to foster community efforts to finance and deliver health services. If there is little or no local tax capacity or responsibility for public expenditure, such efforts may have little success. It is possible that the public finance aspects of community development must be better understood or reformed at a level outside the health sector if efforts within the sector to increase public spending at the community level are to have a reasonable chance of success.

8. Indonesia's 1975 figure is an estimate based on central government spending only; it is unbelievably low and should probably be disregarded.

9. Many European countries now have ratios below 100 people per bed, but such a low ratio is probably not appropriate for the health conditions in most of this sample of countries.

10. See Barnum and Kutzin (1990) and references cited therein.

11. The simple-mindedness of this calculation hardly needs to be explained. Obviously all hospital-related costs should not be assigned to beds. Hospitals deliver many different services, all of which have different costs. The most important distinction lost in these calculations is that between inpatient and outpatient costs. The latter are naively assigned to hospital beds. Despite the simplifying assumptions underlying the analysis, the goal of showing the relative cost of hospitals in terms of local resources merits attention.

12. Korea's figure is misleading because the government owns few hospitals but subsidizes medical bills for the poor, who use both public and private sources of care.

13. Abortion represents 29 percent of admissions under "obstetrical." See appendix table A.18 for details of the subcategories that were aggregated for this table.

14. Malaria is also a leading cause of outpatient visits, which are not counted here. See table 3.13 for information on the causes of death among children in hospitals in Myanmar; they are largely preventable causes.

15. The data presented do not distinguish between the patterns of labor input mixes in the public and private sectors. Rather, they attempt to characterize the aggregate pattern, which may be influenced by broader government policies, including the financing of health education and wage policies for health personnel.

16. The data on health personnel presented in chapter 2 were classified so as to be as comparable as possible across the world. Table 4.13 provides a clearer disaggregation and changes in the supply of physicians and nurses for the early to mid-1980s.

17. Presumably the old figure (for 1981) includes midwives. See the nurse/midwife column.

18. All of the originality in this section was contributed by Jee-Peng Tan, who created table 4.14 and wrote the accompanying discussion.

19. Physicians generally have at least four years of training, nurses about three years, and midwives about two years. The training of lower-level workers is usually counted in weeks or months.

20. The International Comparison Project is a 20-year-old effort to convert national income accounts to a common metric that would allow realistic comparisons across countries. It calculates GNP in terms of real products that take into account the purchasing power of different currencies. The main problem in making GNP comparisons (such as the U.S. dollar comparisons I have been making across countries) is that world prices tend not to apply to untraded goods. In the health sector, this is an important problem. A physician visit in the United States might cost \$50, compared to \$1 for an identical visit (not quality-adjusted) in India. In dollar terms, health spending in India would be counted as one fiftieth of U.S. spending, but the same quantity of services is purchased in both countries. That is the basic problem of converting all expenditures to dollars and comparing them—the comparison

assumes that the price structure is the same as in the United States. That is not the case for developing countries, although it probably is the case for countries at about the same level of GNP as the United States. The International Comparison Project attempts to overcome this problem, essentially by comparing quantities rather than expenditures.

21. As an example of how to read the table, consider the data in the first two rows, showing, respectively, the quantities of medical services consumed per capita, and GDP per capita for 1975 (in real terms). Japan had a per capita GDP that was 68 percent that of the United States, but consumed 84 percent as much medical care.

22. In India, the major exception to this statement, consumption of medical services held steady while output per capita fell relative to the United States.

23. The greater detail corresponds to lower accuracy. These point estimates should be used with caution.

24. The relative price comparisons are somewhat dependent on the base country. In the United States, prices of health services tend to be higher relative to pharmaceuticals and therapeutical goods than in some European countries. For example, if the U.S. ratio is 1:1, the U.K. ratio is 1:1.7. Although using the U.K. ratio as the base would reduce the differences in relative prices between industrial and developing countries, they would still be large for every Asian country examined except Sri Lanka.

25. Koreans behaved in a manner somewhat inconsistent with prices. The price of drugs there is high relative to health services, so the heavy use of pharmaceuticals is unexpected and must result in extremely expensive health care. One suspects that part of the price of drugs may be the services of physicians, but this is true also in India and Thailand, which do not display the same odd demand patterns.

26. Consumption taxes are imposed on alcoholic beverages and cigarettes around the world. They are designed primarily to raise large amounts of revenue through high tax rates on goods for which the price elasticity of demand is low. A secondary justification for these taxes is that they will reduce medically and socially unsound behavior, as determined by those who impose the taxes. Obviously the secondary justification is inconsistent with the primary revenue justification. If consumption is not very sensitive to price, raising the price will not have a strong effect in reducing "sinful" behavior. Not even the most hard-hearted economist has yet proposed such a tax on medical care (also price inelastic) in order to raise revenues or to reduce the incidence of illness. India is at the forefront in this social experiment.

27. Although transportation costs have not been discussed, they are an important cost of many vertical health programs (those that focus on a single service or disease), in the logistics and supervisory operations associated with primary health programs, and in far-flung family planning services. In India, operating costs for transport equipment were 1.16 times the U.S. cost, and communication costs were 1.052 times the U.S. cost (United Nations 1987). With the price of health services standing at 0.09 the U.S. level, it is obvious that the relative cost of extending transport- and supervisory-intensive health programs into peripheral areas in terms of *Indian* prices is quite a different proposition than if *U.S.* prices are used or even if costs are converted to U.S. dollars using the exchange rate.

28. These are not expensive, brand-name drugs but the minimum necessary generic drugs.

5

Mobilizing Nongovernment Resources for Health

This chapter explores the potential for greater use of nontax sources of revenue to support health services in Asia. The importance of these sources stems partially from economic efficiency arguments that justify little role for the government in delivering curative services except on regulatory or redistributive grounds.[1] Nontax resources for health include user fees in the public system, greater reliance on the private sector to deliver curative health services, and insurance coverage to pay catastrophic bills in both the public and the private sectors. The chapter discusses user fees in detail, and provides some information about the current status and prospects for insurance in the region.

User fees

Obviously any discussion of user fees applies only to the public sector; the private sector considers them a necessity, not an optional policy tool. User fees can perform several useful functions in a government health system. They can:

- Increase revenue in the health sector
- Signal to patients that they are consuming valuable resources
- Protect the government from inadvertently subsidizing insurance companies, private physicians, and private patients
- Provide the means for better planning by forcing improved accounting of activities and regular information flows on services delivered
- Profoundly change organizational relationships in centralized systems—where financial flows have historically been from the central administration to facilities, user fee revenues create incentives and resources for decentralized decisionmaking

- Supply an additional policy tool for targeting government subsidies in the health sector to those patients least able to pay.

There are several generic problems with government fee collection systems in the health sector. First, fees are fixed at some point in time and are rarely changed. In Papua New Guinea, for example, fees were set in 1978 and have remained essentially unchanged. The result is a huge deterioration in real terms in the price of the service. A hospital outpatient visit in the public sector costs no more than a soft drink, about $0.50. The *outpatient* fee, which generally includes a free prescription, is less than a third of the cost of a bottle of aspirin or a cold remedy in a private drug store, a fifth or less of the fee charged by traditional healers, and a twentieth or less of the fee charged by private physicians. The public hospital *inpatient* fee, which is about $4.00, represented about 10 percent of the weekly urban minimum wage in 1981 but 8 percent of it in 1987. An inpatient visit is a rare and catastrophic expense for most households (JSI 1990).

Second, fees are often not collected. There are two basic reasons for this. Exemptions from fees are either loosely defined or not carefully applied. In the Philippines, for example, collections in hospitals were less than 10 percent of expenditures in 1987 because 70 percent of the patients were classified as indigent (Asian Development Bank 1987). In India, fees are forgiven for a wide range of people, including civil servants, and collections usually run well below 5 percent of expenditures. The second reason fees are not collected is that facilities often have little incentive to do so. Fee revenues typically are passed on to the central government and have little or no impact on the facility's budget. In Papua New Guinea, the arrangement historically has been to set a target level of fee collections. By regulation, if an institution collects more than its target, some of the excess fee collections could be returned to the facility. In practice, successful fee collecting merely results in a higher goal in subsequent years. Not achieving the goal has had no effect on budget allocations because the facilities must be kept operating (JSI 1990).

A vigorous user fee policy must grapple with these problems. One method is decentralization and autonomy for the more sophisticated institutions. Nepal, for example, has created local governing boards for some of its hospitals and has allowed them to set charges (Asian Development Bank 1987). County hospitals in China are largely self-governing and are expected to recover costs completely. Public hospitals in Korea fully recover costs except for subsidies provided by the state for qualified patients. Public hospitals in Thailand recover a fairly high share of costs but do so primarily through the sale of drugs.

User fee policies in the Asian sample

It is difficult to generalize about user fee policies for some countries, such as India, where policies vary state by state. Other countries, such as Sri Lanka, have national

Table 5.1 Hospital user fee policies in selected Asian countries, late 1980s

Country	*Hospital fee policy*
Bangladesh	Free or nominal
China	Various, prices fixed by state
India	Varies by state, free or nominal for the most part
Indonesia	Detailed fee schedule, low collections
Korea	Full cost recovery from fees, insurance, or state payments for indigents
Malaysia	Detailed fee schedule, low collections
Myanmar	Free
Nepal	Some fees (see text), low collections
Papua New Guinea	Detailed fee schedule, low collections
Philippines	Three-tier fee structure, low collections that declined in the 1980s
Sri Lanka	Free
Thailand	Sale of drugs, relatively high cost recovery (20 to 50 percent of costs)

Note: Low collections means 10 percent or less, usually closer to zero than to 10 percent.
Source: Asian Development Bank 1987.

policies. China has many different types of hospitals with different owners, and cost recovery through fees varies by type of hospital. Table 5.1 contains a recent assessment by each country of its user fee policies, which should be read with these caveats in mind.

Except in China, Korea, and Thailand, fees are not an important source of revenue for curative institutions. Although countries may want to keep fees low for policy reasons, the fact that they are so low in most of the countries means that fees hold great potential as a source of new revenue for systems that need it.

Issues and experience in means testing

Any move toward greater use of fees in the health sector must address the question of how to protect the poor. But it should not be assumed, as it often is, that user charges are inimical to the interests of the poor; in fact, a carefully designed and executed system of user charges can improve the government's ability to target subsidies to those who need them most.

With or without explicit means testing,[2] government spending is targeted to someone. The absence of means testing does not imply that there is no targeting, only that the distributive impact is not explicitly taken into account. As recent investigations of food, health, housing, water, and education subsidies have shown, general price supports may provide some benefits to those who need them most, but benefits are frequently captured by segments of the population who need them least (World Bank 1987b and 1988a). Thus, even if governments do not employ user fees, greater use of means tests would help them target subsidies by better identifying target groups for free services.

A hypothetical example of the equity problem and potential solutions

To become more specific about a typical means testing or poverty alleviation problem in a developing country, take the example of the country shown in table 5.2, which has a population of 100 million and per capita income of $200. It spends $200 million annually, or $2 per capita, to provide free medical services through its system of hospitals, clinics, and rural services (village health workers, an expanded immunization program, health education, a malaria program, and so on). The distribution of expenditure in this table is about what one might expect for the low-income countries in the sample; it is derived roughly from Bangladeshi data. This is the type of distributive information every country should know about its health expenditures but which none in this sample has—hence the hypothetical example. The leading causes of death are infectious diseases, and the infant mortality rate is 100 per thousand live births.

Table 5.2 Hypothetical costs and subsidy patterns

Facility and number of units	*Government cost per beneficiary (U.S. dollars)*	*Number of clients (millions)*	*Total public expenditure (millions of U.S. dollars)*	*Distribution of spending (percent)*	*Average per capita income of clients (U.S. dollars)*	*Average age of client (years)*	*Clients with urban residence (percent)*
Hospital (400 units)	150	0.8	120	60	500	50	80
Clinic (3,000 units)	3	20	60	30	150	40	50
Rural services (20,000 units)	0.50	40	20	10	90	10	10

Source: Author.

The average hospital patient captures $150 of the government's subsidy, clinic patients capture $3, and rural services spend $0.50 per beneficiary. These figures are shown in table 5.2[3] along with other information about the system. In table 5.2, the number of clients reflects the total number of people reached by the unit; for hospitals and clinics it is not meant to reflect total visits. For rural services it is an approximation of the number of beneficiaries of what in many cases are public health interventions.

By any common standard of equity, the subsidy pattern implicit in table 5.2 is awry. It does, however, approximate the distribution of government expenditures for several countries in our sample. Higher-income, older, city-dwelling citizens capture most of the government's health care spending, and this spending is directed to diseases that are treated in hospitals rather than to the primary causes of mortality. The wealthiest 1.3 percent of the population, 80 percent of whom live in the city, capture 60 percent of government spending on health in this example.[4]

Suppose the Ministry of Health decides to transfer $80 million of its hospital subsidy and $30 million of its clinic subsidy to rural services. It does so by charging enough in hospitals to recover $120 per patient and in clinics to recover $2 per patient. The charges allow hospitals and clinics to continue to operate at the current level even though the government has transferred its tax revenue to rural health services.

As far as targeting is concerned, and given our minimal information about the clients, this reallocation of the subsidy improves equity significantly. When the fees are introduced, however, the ministry must figure out how to forgive fees for hospital and clinic patients who cannot pay them. Hospitals will now have a subsidy of $40 million, and clinics a subsidy of $10 million, to distribute to the needy.

Assuming that there is no insurance and all hospital expenses will be out-of-pocket, there are many options for targeting the remaining subsidy. If there is health insurance, the menu of options expands. Listed below are some of the alternatives available to the ministry.[5]

Administratively inexpensive measures.

- *General price subsidy continued.* The general price subsidy could be continued by subsidizing each hospital patient by $30 and each clinic patient by $1. That would not assist the poor who cannot afford the fee in the first place.
- *General price subsidy geographically targeted.* The general price subsidy could be continued only in rural hospitals and clinics, which might be enough to maintain free services there. That tactic would reach many people in rural areas who could pay and miss many people in cities who are poor, but it would target generally poorer areas.
- *Targeting by age.* Free services could be provided only for people younger than 5 and older than 70.
- *Targeting by catastrophic medical events.* All patients could be required to pay for a minimum number of days of inpatient care, but beyond this minimum length of stay, out-of-pocket expenses would decline or stop. Alternatively, the stopping point could be keyed to the bill that accumulates. This approach ties the means test to the illness episode itself and thus provides a form of catastrophic or stop-loss insurance. Outpatient visits would not be subsidized. This approach is not directly targeted to the poor but emphasizes the insurance problem related to inpatient stays.
- *Targeting by self-selection/price discrimination.* The hospital could provide different levels of inpatient services that are clinically equivalent but have different amenities. For example, private rooms with a bath, air conditioning, and choice of attending physician could be priced substantially above cost. Use of the outpatient

department could also be priced above cost, because people have the option of using less costly clinics. These profitable services would, along with the central government subsidies, be used to maintain general price supports for inpatients choosing wards. Under this approach, the client determines the tradeoffs between paying and using the charity ward. Although many countries provide services in "pay" wards, they are often so heavily subsidized that they have perverse equity effects. A limiting factor in this scenario is whether pricing the higher-amenity services well above cost would drive away too many patients and thus prevent making a profit on those services.

Administratively costly measures.

• *Sliding fee system with social worker verification.* Patients requesting assistance from the hospital with their fees would be interviewed by social workers, who would certify their eligibility. Such interviews would collect information about the client that could be subsequently verified. The more detailed the information and the greater the verification requirement, the more expensive the system. Suppose this approach required 1,000 social workers plus procedures and bookkeeping devices that used up 10 percent of the free care subsidy for administration. For this approach to be preferred to one of the costless techniques, it would have to achieve significantly better targeting. In other words, if the social worker approach tended to award subsidies only to children under 5 and to the elderly over 70, there is no reason to prefer it to the age criterion. If it added a few people between 5 and 70, the question would be whether diverting 10 percent of the budget to achieve that improvement in targeting would be worth the cost. The 10 percent administrative cost could be allocated instead to supplement the age criterion with a catastrophic subsidy for the period of middle age, which might solve the same problem without an additional administrative cost.

• *Central certification system.* The ministry could require all patients to register formally each year, providing complete information about the household. Each household would be given a card entitling it to a specific fee reduction (based on sliding fee scales) for different hospital services. Alternatively, people could purchase vouchers whose prices would be prorated by income, with the price determined by social workers' evaluations. The administrative cost of this centralized approach would presumably be higher than that of performing the certification at the point of purchase, but leakages might be reduced by greater enforcement capabilities on the part of the central government as well as the requirement that the determination of poverty be made outside the health system (when people are healthy). It is more difficult to certify the indigent during a hospital emergency. One possible advantage of this more bureaucratic approach is that there may be economies of scale in using a standardized method for all subsidy programs. Korea uses an approach somewhat along these lines.

• *Geographic poverty profiles and subsidized facilities.* Sample surveys could identify pockets of poverty where a general price subsidy in a specific facility (without targeting among patients in the facility) would reach the poor with few leakages. The location of the subsidized facilities would target the subsidy. This approach differs from the costless rural subsidy described earlier because it requires ranking geographic areas by average need. Although this would require some additional expenditure, it would probably be less costly than other methods discussed in this section. It would also be more applicable to clinics, which have a more localized service area than hospitals.

In principle, the costs of each approach could be determined relative to its effectiveness as a targeting mechanism. The obvious tradeoff for each method is between the cost of the test and the amount of leakage it allows.[6] Many of the methods outlined above are feasible in even the poorest countries. When the question of user fees and means testing arises, it is often automatically assumed that a large administrative structure is necessary to certify the indigent. The cost of such a structure must be weighed against the cost of leakages associated with less expensive methods that might effectively achieve the desired results.

Self-selection criteria are particularly attractive because they not only minimize administrative costs, they also expand the choices available to consumers. These mechanisms also give consumers an incentive to reveal their willingness to pay, which is the opposite of an administrative approach in which they are given incentives to appear as poor as possible. In any self-selection approach, the larger the menu of choices, the better it is likely to work for both clients and administrators.

What this list of options makes clear is that there are so many ways to target subsidies that governments could probably do better in targeting public subsidies by using one or more of these devices in combination with user fees than by using a blanket zero-price policy, as most in this Asian sample effectively do today.

Methods used in the Asian sample to target health care subsidies

Means tests must have goals. Policymakers must determine what should be identified by the means test—long-term deprivation, short-term acute shortfalls in income, or people who simply cannot care for themselves. Many different filters are applied in the world, including geography, diseases, age, nutritional status, seasonal/geographic interactions, village elder certification, asset ownership, income, and self-selection. All approaches attempt to identify poor groups, but some are aimed more exclusively at conditions, diseases, or age groups that have policy significance for reasons other than income alone.

India: Facility-based determinations. In India, government policies on cost recovery vary by state, although it is safe to say that only a small percentage of costs is recovered through fees. A study in Maharashtra State found that exemptions from charges in public hospitals and dispensaries were clearly set down by regulation. A peculiar combination of people has been exempted from most fees, with the poor being only one of those groups. Those with incomes of less than 180 rupees (Rs.) per month in urban areas (Rs. 150 in rural areas), civil servants and their families, medical and nursing staff, and medical students do not have to pay at all. Three other income categories are defined: in urban areas, Rs. 151–300 per month, Rs. 301–500 per month, and Rs. 500+ per month. A full list of charges is published for each class, but there are no charges for immunizations and most maternal and child health services. Despite the apparent completeness of the scheme, hospitals collected less than one percent of costs in 1984–85. The reason is that the system depends on self-declaration of income, and almost everyone declares that they earn less than Rs. 180 per month.

A 1986 study of eight community health projects in India sponsored by nongovernmental organizations found that most charged user fees for drugs or services and two charged a membership fee. All of the projects charged according to ability to pay. One of the projects with a membership fee charged a minimum annual fee of Rs. 12 for those with a monthly income below Rs. 300, and an annual fee of up to Rs. 300 for households with monthly incomes of Rs. 2,500 or more. The second membership-based project charged Rs. 1 per month or Rs. 10 per year, but 20 percent of the members were excused from paying. Another project relied on the doctors' judgments of the clients' ability to pay (Elkins and others 1986, and Indian Institute of Management 1987).

Indonesia: Village headman/council. In Indonesia, a full set of tariffs has been developed for every level of government health facility and every type of service. Prices for outpatient visits for four classes of patients range from 20 to 50 percent of the Drug Price Index. Inpatient days are charged for five different classes, ranging from 1.5 to 13 times the Food Price Index. In one Jakarta hospital in 1987, these rates corresponded to $0.30 for an outpatient visit (apparently for any class), $0.36 per day for the lowest class of inpatient care, and $18.50 per day, plus the cost of drugs, for the "VIP class." Outpatient fees for health centers range from $0.18 to $0.61.

The poor are protected in this system by the low fees for outpatient and inpatient care in the lowest class of service. Assuming an actual cost per visit of 800 rupiah and two outpatient visits per person per year, the cost would be no more than 3 percent of average rural income per capita. In addition, the local village chief or other authorized official can issue an affidavit of indigence that formally excuses all fees for the recipient. These certificates are apparently quite easy to obtain. Hospitals in 1986 recovered about 20 percent of their costs, and health centers recovered only 3 percent, according to an internal World Bank report.

Korea: Central certification system. Korea is a special case: its health care is delivered primarily through the private sector, and government hospitals are organized as public corporations that recover most of their costs from fees. Private clinics and hospitals account for about 95 percent of all medical facilities, and employ 72 percent of the physicians and contain 72 percent of hospital beds. From 1961 to 1976, free treatment was provided for the poor directly through government facilities. In 1977 the Medical Care Assistance Program was established to help pay the medical bills of the poor, who are divided into three categories.

Indigents, or first-class beneficiaries, are defined as those with no means of support, such as the chronically ill and people living in public facilities. By definition they are easy to identify. Second-class beneficiaries are those who have no steady income and rely on public assistance. In 1986 those whose monthly income was less than 42,000 won ($50) in large cities, 38,000 won in other cities, and 34,000 won in rural areas qualified for public assistance. The third class consists of those who do not qualify for public assistance but meet less stringent income or asset criteria for assistance with medical bills only.

In 1985, 643,000 first-class beneficiaries (1.5 percent of the population) were eligible for free inpatient and outpatient care, although the total number of visits and hospital days was limited. There were 1,819,000 second-class beneficiaries (4.4 percent of the population) who were eligible for a 50 percent subsidy on *inpatient* costs if they lived in a major city, an 80 percent subsidy if they lived elsewhere, and free *outpatient* care no matter where they lived. The third category (medical assistance) contained nearly 2 million beneficiaries (5 percent of the population) in 1986. They qualified for a 40 percent subsidy on inpatient care in major cities and 60 percent elsewhere, and a 33 percent subsidy on outpatient care. For the portion of inpatient care not paid for by the government, zero-interest loans were available. These three groups accounted for about 11 percent of the population in 1986.

Government hospitals are used extensively for inpatient treatment under this program, but private physicians are enlisted to provide outpatient care, for which they receive fees estimated to be about half the market rate. Thus the government subsidizes medical care for the indigent but expects private practitioners to contribute as well. A recent development in Korea is the extension of insurance coverage to 100 percent of the population, but that is unlikely to change the government's role in paying for care that it currently funds under this program. It is expected that coverage under the Medical Assistance Program will be expanded to 15 to 16 percent of the population, who will not be required to pay insurance premiums (Park and Yeon 1981; Yeon 1985; Republic of Korea, Economic Planning Department 1986; Lee 1987; and Kim 1987).

Malaysia: Facility-based determinations. In Malaysia, user charges for outpatient care are about $0.24 for general outpatient services and $2.08 for specialist outpatient care. There are three classes of inpatient charges. Those unable to pay must request an exemption, and they are interviewed to assess their ability to pay. Apparently they are quite convincing; in recent years revenues from hospital charges have amounted to only 5 percent of government expenditures (Ghazali, Salam, and Baba 1987).

Papua New Guinea: Facility-based determinations. In Papua New Guinea, outpatient visits in hospitals cost K 0.50, and inpatient care costs K 4.00 for any length of stay. Exceptions for hospital fees are provided for children under age 12, people over age 60, and cases of sexually transmitted diseases. Eligibility is determined by the clerk at the entrance to the hospital. Despite the formal aspects of this approach, it is almost completely porous, with no hospitals collecting more than 5 percent of their expenditures at present. Papua New Guinea plans to cross subsidize within hospitals by charging higher prices in intermediate wards and for specialist outpatient visits. These high prices would subsidize much lower prices in wards and for regular outpatient care. Papua New Guinea will probably have some trouble succeeding with the plan, however. Intermediate ward services are poor, and it is not clear that the patient gets a significantly better service for a steeply higher price. As a result, occupancy rates are low in the intermediate wards of most hospitals. Patients in the intermediate wards currently receive approximately the same daily subsidy as do patients in the public wards (Thomason and others 1987).

Philippines: Facility-based determinations. In the Philippines, there are three different levels of service in government hospitals. Class A patients pay the full cost of care based on Medicare-reimbursable prices.[7] Class B patients pay at least 50 percent of those prices. Class C patients pay what they can. Class D patients receive free care. Medical social workers interview patients to determine their ability to pay. In 1979, 65 percent of the patients in government hospitals were class C or D patients, 13 percent were class A or B patients, and 22 percent were class A patients with Medicare coverage. Private hospitals in 1980 had the following pattern of inpatients: 7 percent indigents, 39 percent self-pay, and 54 percent Medicare.

A 1985 study of 60 district hospitals in all regions except Manila showed that 72 percent of patients were declared indigent. In 1985 operating income from all government health services was only 4.6 percent of expenditures, but hospitals collected about 10 percent of their costs (according to an internal World Bank report, and Integrated Health Care Services 1987), presumably in large part from Medicare reimbursements.

Singapore: Price discrimination in hospitals. In Singapore, there are five classes of wards in public hospitals (table 5.3). The subsidy pattern, except for class B1 services, reflects an effort to provide the bulk of government subsidies to people who are most sensitive to prices. In 1981 about 80 percent of patients chose class C accommodations, so the subsidy in effect goes to a large share of the population and is not particularly sensitive to poverty. Roughly a fifth of the Ministry of Health's

Table 5.3 Classes of hospital services in Singapore

Class	*Level of privacy (number of beds)*	*Costs covered by the fee (percent)*	*Amenity: Choice of doctor*
A1	1	100	Choose doctor
A2	2	100	Choose doctor
B1	6	15	Choose doctor
B2	8-10	75	Assigned doctor
C	Open ward	25	Assigned doctor

Source: Westinghouse Health Systems and Government of Malaysia 1985.

budget is covered by fees (Westinghouse Health Systems and Government of Malaysia 1985).

Thailand: Central certification system. In Thailand there are no professional fees in government hospitals, yet hospitals recover nearly half their costs through charges for drugs, tests, procedures, and room and board. Thailand has a formal Free Medical Care Project, started in 1975, under which indigents receive free care. Until 1980 the head of the health facility decided who would qualify for free services. After 1980 free medical care cards were issued to single people with monthly incomes of less than $66 and to families with monthly incomes of less than $87. The card must be renewed every three years. In 1985 about 20 percent of the population, or 11 million people, held cards.

The program receives a separate allocation that is distributed to government health units to defray the costs of providing free care to card holders. In 1986 the total cost was $26.25 million. The Ministry of Health budget in 1985 was $645 million. It is estimated that hospitals provide twice the amount of free services that would be accounted for only by card holders, so there are additional informal subsidies being provided to people who do not hold cards (Myers, Mongkolsmai, and Causino 1985 and Wibulpolprasert, Buapradubkul, and Chantrasatid 1987).

Methods not commonly used in the Asian sample to target health care subsidies

One short-hand method for means testing or targeting nutrition and health programs for children and mothers is monitoring children's growth, both a health intervention and a financial screening device. The nutritional status of children has been repeatedly found to be strongly associated with income and landholdings in developing countries. A recent study in Nepal, for example, found that measures of stunting (height for age), wastage (weight for height), and weight for age worsened significantly as the proxy for household income—the value of crops produced by the household—declined (Martorell, Leslie, and Moock 1984). Stewart (1987) suggests that measures of malnutrition, including those already identified, as well as hospital statistics on the incidence of kwashiorkor, marasmus, and low birth weight are excellent indicators of severe economic stress in a population.

Pregnancy, malnourished children, infectious diseases, immunizations, and diarrhea are a few of the many physical conditions that are targeted for free or subsidized interventions in developing countries. Any malnutrition-based subsidy for poor households is almost certainly well targeted, because most poverty lines are linked to food expenditures.

Insurance and risk-sharing mechanisms

There is enormous confusion about the potential for health insurance in developing countries: whether it might have any positive equity effects, whether it would enhance or reduce efficiency in the sector, and why governments should be interested in it at all. Box 5.1 provides, through an example, some of the basic logic behind health insurance. The logic is powerful, and insurance has proved to be a useful financial tool in the health sector in most of the industrial countries and many middle-income countries, especially in Latin America. In this sample, it constitutes an important element of the financing strategies of only two countries, China and Korea. There is no question that the problems associated with insurance, including administrative costs, moral hazard, adverse selection, and incentives for price escalation, are serious. They will slow the spread of insurance to the poorer, more rural countries; and the problems with insurance may lead some governments to substitute public services and rationing mechanisms for it.

Box 5.1 Insurance, adverse selection, moral hazard, and cost escalation

Suppose everyone from age 10 to age 60 has a 1 in 10,000 chance of experiencing a $5,000 hospital bill in any given year. Each person's expected loss in 1989 is (0.0001) X ($5,000) = $0.50. A risk-averse individual would be willing to pay more than $0.50 for insurance that prevents the loss, which would transform the low-probability but immense loss into a certain but minuscule loss.

If an insurance company could assemble 10,000 people with this loss probability and collect $0.50 from each of them, it could expect to incur one $5,000 loss a year and would just break even if it had no administrative costs. If each person would pay $1.00 a year to avoid the loss, which seems likely, the insurance company could probably make a tidy profit, assuming it could assemble the risk pool at low cost. This is the definition of a catastrophic loss: a low-probability, catastrophic event. Clearly such a loss is fairly easy to insure against. In fact, the attractiveness of insurance is that the more horrendous the loss, the more likely it is that a person can protect himself or herself from it as long as it is a low-probability loss (if such losses are not low-probability events, humans will soon join the dinosaurs).

Compare to this scenario a small but high-probability loss, such as dental checkups. Suppose a person has a 95 percent chance of spending $100 a year on dental care. A risk-averse person might be willing to spend more than $95 for dental insurance (but not more than $100). Unless the insurance company could provide dental insurance with an administrative cost below $5, dental checkups would be an uninsurable loss. To the insurance company, there is little chance of a profit; to the purchaser, the insurance component is nil. It is for all practical purposes a forced savings plan. Similarly, if an individual at age 85 has an 80 percent chance of a $5,000 hospital bill, the insurance premium would be punitive and unlikely to be preferred to the loss. Thus, even a catastrophic loss can become an uninsurable event; it all depends on the probability of the loss.

"Saving for a rainy day" is not an economically efficient substitute for insurance. A person with a low-probability expected loss of $5,000 could put $100 a year for 50 years under the mattress and finally achieve (at the end of life) the protection that would otherwise have been available every year by buying our insurance plan for $1.00 a year

Box 5.1 Insurance, adverse selection, moral hazard, and cost escalation (cont.)

for a total lifetime premium of only $50.00. The efficiency gains due to insurance are obvious. There is no alternative to the pooling of risks that provides the same level of protection.

Insurance creates three problems by creating incentives for consumers and providers to behave in ways that, if uncontrolled, would destroy the insurance system: adverse selection, moral hazard, and incentives for cost escalation. Adverse selection intrudes when people with a high probability of a loss systematically join the plan while those with a low probability of a loss do not join. In our example, suppose the insurance pool is comprised of people with a 1/100 chance of a loss. If the insurance company calculates the premium on the assumption that the pool has a 1/10,000 probability of a loss, it will lose $490,000 if the premium is $1.00 a year. The least expensive correction is to use the police power of the state to force groups randomly selected on health status, such as workers, to participate in the insurance plan. The most expensive correction would be for the state to do nothing, because then the insurance company would be forced (at the limit) to physically examine all potential beneficiaries to ascertain independently their riskiness. Insurance companies have other less costly methods at their disposal, but every alternative is costly.

Moral hazard means that the probability of a loss rises as a result of joining the insurance scheme. A person's probability of a loss may increase from 1/10,000 to 1/9,000 after he joins the insurance plan because he is no longer so fearful of the loss. If that happens, our insurance plan will have expected losses of $5,556 instead of $5,000. The extra $556 is caused by behavior changes precipitated by insurance coverage. Moral hazard can be reduced by forcing clients to pay part of the costs of their care before insurance takes over.

Consumers, but especially physicians, can create pressures for costs to escalate. They do so by increasing both the probability and the cost of a loss. A 100 percent increase in the cost will raise the premium in this example to only $2.00, so insurance companies will find little support among their clients for their efforts to control the cost of physicians' healing behavior.

Insurance has gotten a bit of a bad name in developing countries because donors have supported rural insurance plans that cover all problems (including a large share of uninsurable losses), that depend on voluntary membership (no protection against adverse selection), that have no copayments or deductibles (encouraging moral hazard), and that contain no clear mechanism for collecting premiums regularly. Even the famous health card system in Thailand has most of these problems (see Asian Development Bank 1987 for a description of the Thai plan).

The main lesson of this primer is that catastrophic losses are the easiest and cheapest to insure against. That is the place to start in creating insurance plans in developing countries. This idea fits well with the problem of financing hospitals because hospitals are where catastrophic losses take place, which is hard on patients and destroys the financial viability of hospitals.

Table 5.4 Coverage and facility ownership of insurance plans in selected Asian countries, mid-1980s

Country	*Plan*	*Facilities owned*	*Coverage*
Bangladesh	Government	no	medical allowance for civil servants
China	GEIS	no	civil servants, students
	Labor insurance		
	State enterprise	no	enterprise, industrial, mine workers
	Town and village enterprises	no	enterprise, industrial, mine workers
	Private	no	private enterprises, contract workers
	Collective	no	rural townships and villages
India	CGHS	..	civil servants
	ESIS	yes	industrial
	NICL	no	Mediclaim—privately purchased
	Rural	..	cooperatives
Indonesia	ASKES	no	civil servants
	ASTEK	no	industrial accidents
	PKTK (or DUKM)		
	Dana Sehat	no	rural
Korea	Industrial	no	labor
	KMIC	no	civil servants, teachers
	Occupational	no	self-employed
	Regional	no	rural
	Medical Aid	no	uninsured who qualify for assistance
Malaysia	SOCSO	no	formally employed (with wage ceiling)
	EPF	no	forced savings plan for employees
	Private	no	65 private insurance companies
Myanmar	Social Security	no	public (83 percent) and private industrial workers
Nepal	Informal	yes	some pilot schemes in rural areas
Papua New Guinea	Public Service Assoc.	no	association members
Philippines	GSIS	no	civil servants; other employed; self-employed
	SSS	no	voluntary
	Private/firm	..	private sector insurance plans
Sri Lanka	NIC and ICSL	no	government insurance companies
	Private	..	some private plans
Thailand	Workmen's comp.	no	firms of >20 employees, selected provinces
	Private insurance	no	21 private insurance companies
	Rural	no	health card funds
	Government	no	civil servants
	Public enterprise	no	employees of public enterprises
	Free care	no	certified indigents

.. Not available.

Source: Same as for appendix table A.17.

Patterns of coverage and expenditure

Available information on insurance is, to say the least, sketchy. Table 5.4 gives the names and coverage of the known insurance plans in the sample of Asian countries. In contrast to Latin America, most of the insurance schemes do not own their own facilities.

Neither Bangladesh nor Nepal has a formal health insurance plan. Both provide government employees with small medical allowances that have basically no insurance value.

For another segment of the sample, insurance plans are limited to worker compensation schemes that do not really cover medical problems, except those related to accidents in the workplace. This type of insurance is the primary approach used in Indonesia, Myanmar, and Thailand. Malaysia, which follows the same pattern, and Sri Lanka also provide public insurance through their free public medical systems. China, India, Korea, and the Philippines have larger general-purpose health insurance plans that vary substantially in character.

Figure 5.1 reproduces information from chapter 4 to show the estimated contribution of insurance and out-of-pocket spending to total expenditure in each country for 1986 or 1987. For countries that currently have a small contribution from insurance, but a relatively large contribution from out-of-pocket spending (India, Indonesia, the Philippines, and Thailand), there are incentives to rely much more on insurance

Figure 5.1 Share of health spending by government, private sources, and insurance in selected Asian countries, most recent year

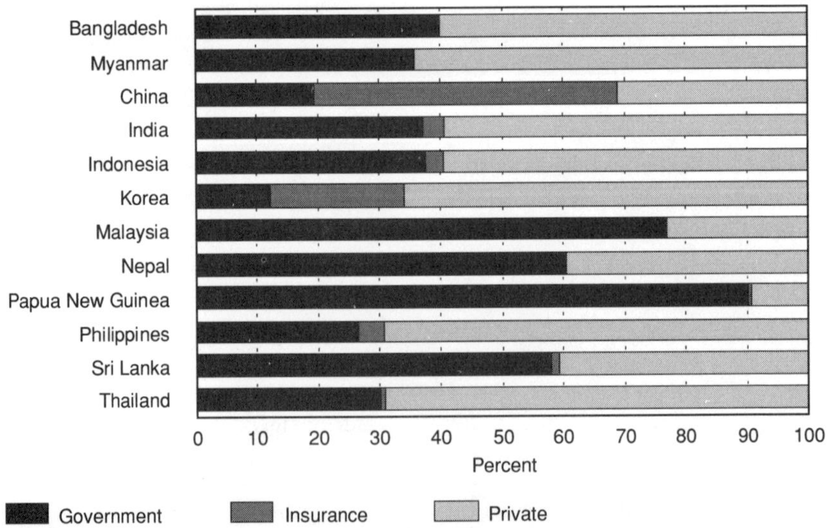

Source: Appendix table A.13.

financing in the future. The share of expenditure financed by insurance in Korea is also likely to increase—and has probably increased substantially already—because that country has established a plan to move toward 100 percent coverage of the population over the last two years. Countries that currently have little or no insurance coverage but high private spending (Bangladesh, Malaysia, Myanmar, and Sri Lanka) could reduce the burden of private spending by exploring policy options for greater insurance coverage.

How do these spending levels correspond to coverage? Figure 5.2 shows the best estimate that could be developed of the coverage of nonagricultural workers and the population as a whole for the Asian sample. China, Korea, and the Philippines have relatively high coverage, with China reaching nearly 90 percent of nonagricultural labor through insurance. The remainder of the sample covers 10 percent or less of the formal sector labor force, which typically corresponds to a smaller percentage of the entire population.

For Korea and the Philippines—countries with relatively high coverage but a low proportion of spending from insurance (and high private expenditure)—insurance probably covers a limited set of risks or has payment caps. In Korea, for example, private spending is $98 per capita but insurance spending is only $58 per beneficiary, suggesting very limited benefits. In the Philippines, private spending is $9 per capita, while the insurance funds spend less than $2 per beneficiary. In contrast, private

Figure 5.2 Percentage of workers and population covered by health insurance in selected Asian countries, 1986-87
(estimated)

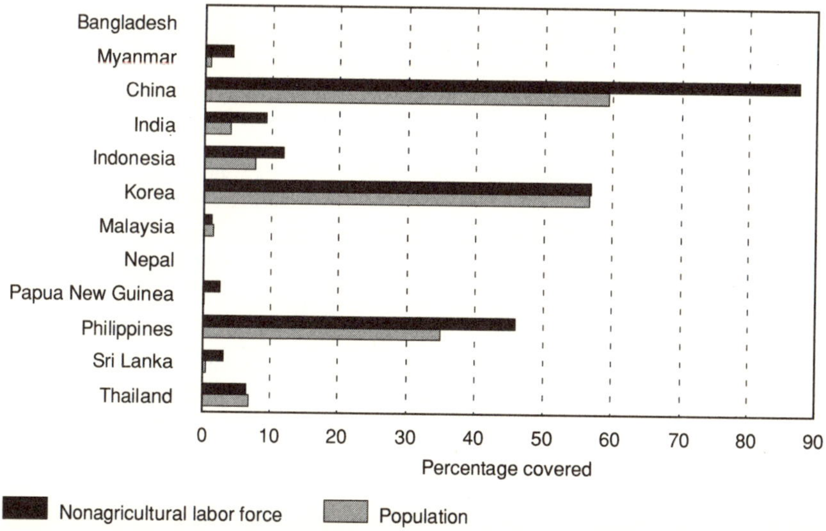

Source: Appendix table A.16.

spending in China is about $3 per capita but insurance spends about $9 per beneficiary—suggesting that the wide coverage of insurance plans is coupled with substantial benefits. A different pattern holds in several countries that have limited insurance coverage—few are covered by insurance, but their benefits are relatively generous. In India, for example, private spending per capita is about $7, but the insurance spends about $12 per beneficiary.[8]

This limited information suggests that countries could profit from examining detailed information about insurance coverage and benefits. An insurance system with broad coverage and reasonable benefits can have an equity-improving effect for the large segment of the population that is covered, because benefits are usually tied to need rather than to income.[9] But small plans with narrow coverage of high-income segments of the population tend to reinforce inequities, especially if they receive public subsidies. In small plans such as in India or Indonesia, a narrow slice of the population receives benefits substantially higher than those available to everyone else through the public health system.

Is health insurance a sensible financing policy even for poor countries?

The simple answer to this question is that we do not know. We do know that it is feasible, and that it can allow the government to target more central spending to public health activities. China has shown that insurance can provide half of the health sector's revenues even at an extremely low level of per capita income. Insurance is widespread even in rural areas. Although rural plans collapsed in the late 1970s and early 1980s with the responsibility system, they appear to have rebounded as institutional structures became more regularized and government policy adapted to the changes by the mid-1980s. Rural and private sector insurance are now the fastest growing areas of insurance coverage in China, according to an internal World Bank report.

Insurance is not an activity that can start from the bottom up. If coverage does not begin in the formal sector, there is a high probability that the plan will be made infeasible by moral hazard, high administrative costs, and adverse selection. Rural areas can be covered, as China has shown, but institutional structures must first be identified to which a rural plan could be tied (such as farmers' organizations for irrigation or credit, marketing cooperatives, or even churches). Because of the institutional and economic requirements of insurance, it is probably most feasible to start in cities and expand outward.

Insurance has several benefits for even the poorest countries. First, it allows the government to diversify the sources of revenue for the health sector. Second, in a country such as Bangladesh, where there is little or no formal insurance, it gives the segment of the population most able to pay the opportunity to pay for their own health care. In Bangladesh, converting the medical allowance to an insurance premium for civil servants would give them an improved benefit and allow the government to reduce free care from public hospitals for that segment of the population. Third, it provides a payment mechanism that is necessary for greater private sector involvement in providing curative care. If countries value any of these characteristics of insurance, they could benefit from it.

A common argument against insurance is that poorer countries cannot afford a reasonable benefits package. That is simply untrue. If, as discussed in box 5.1, a plan covers only catastrophic illness, it should be inexpensive. The following example from Sri Lanka provides a clearer idea of the issues involved in planning and costing out an insurance system.

In 1986 there were two insurance companies in Sri Lanka, both government-owned, that sold group health insurance. The most expensive plan covered surgical and hospital expenses up to $1,419 a year and cost a family of four $135. The least expensive plan covered surgical and hospital expenses up to $160 a year at a rate of $13 a year for a family of four. The most expensive policy paid up to $14 a day for room and board; the least expensive, $1.24. The least expensive policy would have cost less than one percent of average income for a family of four in 1986 and would have covered all costs in Sri Jayewardenepura Hospital, an independent government-owned hospital (a parastatal), except part of room and board. The annual cost of the least expensive insurance policy in 1986 was a third of per capita health spending (government plus private). There is so little health insurance in Sri Lanka that the costs of providing this coverage would probably fall as coverage widened because of the high fixed costs of administering even a small plan. Catastrophic health insurance on a much larger scale may be feasible if these figures are accurate.

The foregoing information on insurance plans suggests a striking divergence of experience with insurance in the region. China is probably the country with the longest experience in creating and administering third-party payment mechanisms on a large scale. India's public insurance system, covering only about 4 percent of the population, has been in existence since 1952, however, and its small relative size translates into a huge operation that covers 28 million people, owns a large physical plant, and employs thousands. The system is larger than many national systems in Latin America. There is considerable interest in all countries in this sample in expanding insurance coverage. It will be one of the major policy issues of the next decade.

Conclusion

Countries in Asia rely on various strategies to mobilize nontax resources for health, including charging fees for public services, relying on private sector delivery, and using insurance coverage. The data and discussion suggest several broad policy directions.

In the more *revenue-constrained* countries, such as Bangladesh and Nepal, which would clearly benefit from higher spending on health and the diversion of public resources from curative services, user fees may provide an attractive alternative to 100 percent government financing of the state health system. Because of the high incidence of poverty, any such fee strategy would require careful targeting of the remaining government subsidies to the neediest. Furthermore, greater dependence on the private sector and private-public partnerships to deliver care holds great potential for improving the operational efficiency of the health systems in those countries. That is particularly true in Bangladesh, which is training large numbers of physicians that the public sector cannot employ.[10] Insurance is not an important option for either country, although insurance for formal sector employees (especially government employees) would start the development of the necessary institutional structures and create a mechanism through which those who are best off pay for their own health care. Both countries already pay their public employees a small medical allowance; on efficiency grounds alone, it would make considerably more sense to turn the allowance into an insurance premium (see box 5.1 for an elaboration of the logic underlying this statement).

The Philippines could also be considered a revenue-constrained country because of its low public spending on health. Its private sector is well developed, while its public sector invests heavily in hospitals despite the relatively low public sector spending. In that country, a combination of greater cost recovery, less duplication of private sector activities, and greater attention to the moribund national insurance system would increase economic efficiency in the sector and allow the government to retarget its expenditures. It may be less important in the Philippines to increase public spending than it is to use it more effectively. Because of its level of development, it has many options available to accomplish that goal. Indonesia is a similar case, although its insurance systems are not as well developed.

Countries with *relatively high private and public spending*, which include India, Myanmar, and Thailand, are less constrained and may have little interest in adjusting their policies. The development of insurance in those countries is probably desirable from the client's viewpoint, however, given the countries' current high private expenditure. Greater attention to insurance is also sensible on grounds of public welfare, because these are the countries in which disease patterns are likely to change rapidly in the future, leading to greater demands for chronic care and the expensive hospital-based technologies that it requires. In each country, the government remains heavily involved in the provision of hospital services, which insurance is best suited to finance.

Three countries, Malaysia, Papua New Guinea, and, to a lesser degree, Sri Lanka, have *high total expenditure on health that comes largely from the public sector*. Such expenditure patterns may be the result of carefully considered decisions and government priorities in those countries; thus, there may be little desire or felt need to change the sources of revenue. But there is little question, given the experience of the other countries in the sample, that some portion of the high public expenditure does little more than substitute for private expenditure that would be made anyway, either out of pocket or through insurance. Because these countries have exceptionally high spending, there is wide scope (economically, if perhaps not politically) for adjustments in how the sector is financed and how carefully the government targets its own spending.

Finally, China and Korea have *high total expenditure, low direct government expenditure, and relatively heavy dependence on insurance financing*. They are rapidly moving into the policy problems associated with the health sector in industrial countries—cost containment, rationing of medical care, optimal reimbursement methods, and ways to plan better for health sector investments under decentralized third-party payment systems. These issues are not discussed in this report but have been covered extensively elsewhere.

Notes

1. These issues are discussed clearly and in more detail in World Bank 1987b.

2. *Means testing* refers to the generic question of determining who is poor and therefore eligible for a subsidy.

3. The allocation of the budget in table 5.2 is fairly typical of the poorest countries. However, the distribution by income, age, and urban or rural residence is a guess about what a typical situation might look like.

4. In this and subsequent sections the discussion of subsidies, as they are called here, or who captures government spending, may refer to rural and urban differences. To some extent this approach creates a straw man. It does not make sense on efficiency grounds to locate major hospitals in rural areas, so hospital spending alone will tend to skew the distribution of public expenditure to cities. On the other hand, if the poor are predominantly in the countryside, and because they are the ones plagued by the diseases of poverty, spending public money on urban hospitals does them little good. Even if hospitals are located in cities, governments can do something about the implicit diversion of funds to support them by encouraging hospitals to pay their own way.

5. All of these methods assume that the ministry has a fixed budget within which it must attempt to meet its subsidy goals. Thus the amount of the subsidy and eligibility are both contingent on the available budget. This approach contrasts with an alternative in which eligibility is not contingent on the size of the budget; instead, the budget is contingent on the number of eligible people and the desired subsidy level. The second approach is rarely used because it means governments are willing to pay whatever it takes to reach poverty alleviation goals.

6. This orientation to preventing leakages to the nonpoor does not address the opposite problem, the effect of the means test's missing people who are poor.

7. Medicare is the national health insurance program, which sets reimbursement levels for its beneficiaries for all types of inpatient service.

8. Appendix table A.17 contains a summary of the benefits and coverage of existing insurance plans.

9. This statement would not be true if different types of workers were covered under many different schemes with different benefits.

10. Given the personnel ratios in Bangladesh, and the constrained budgets, an argument might be made that the government service should not employ more physicians. But no such statement can be made without better understanding the relative costs of physicians and other personnel.

6

Patterns in the Targeting of Government Expenditure

In most countries the government or an agency of the government is the single largest spending authority in the health sector. Where spending comes from several levels of government or from multiple spending agencies within a government, this authority may be fragmented. Nevertheless, the allocation of public health resources has a significant effect on the overall efficiency and equity of health sector spending.

The previous chapter documented methods of means testing that governments have relied on to target subsidies to individuals. This chapter focuses on the outcomes of these and other targeting efforts, as revealed in the broad patterns of allocation by health criteria and population groups. Two issues are especially important. First, to what extent is public expenditure targeted to address health problems whose mitigation would generate benefits beyond individuals? And second, to what extent is spending targeted to socially disadvantaged population groups who might consume fewer health services than socially optimal if they had to bear the full cost of those services?

Detailed data to document these issues are not available in a comparable form for all countries in this study. However, some insights emerge from piecing together aggregate data for selected Asian countries, including India, Indonesia, Malaysia, Papua New Guinea, and Bangladesh.

Public health expenditure in India

India uses two budgets, one to implement new programs according to the current five-year plan ("plan" expenditure) and the other to fund recurrent costs for continuing programs ("nonplan" expenditure). Plan expenditure is not strictly capital expenditure because it also includes spending on recurrent costs of new programs that have not yet been moved into the regular budget. In this section, data from 16 states containing 95 percent of India's population are used to analyze the distribution of plan and nonplan expenditure on health and family welfare in 1982–83. State-level expenditure is the basis of the cross-state analysis. Central expenditure cannot be broken down by state, so it is not possible to analyze directly how it offsets or reinforces state spending patterns. But because central spending accounted for only 14 percent of total spending on health in 1983 for these states and because other approaches are used to infer the likely effect of central spending, the lack of data on central spending by state may not be as large a problem as it would first appear.

Patterns of state allocations

State-level data on infant mortality rates, per capita incomes, and per capita health expenditure are displayed in table 6.1.[1] The simple relation between state income and spending per capita is shown in figure 6.1. As might be expected, states with higher incomes tend to spend more on health and family welfare, but the relation between income and spending is weak. The range in total spending is large. Himachal Pradesh, with per capita income of 2,230 rupees, spends the most, nearly five times more per person than Bihar, with per capita income of 1,174 rupees. If the three states with high per capita incomes but low health spending are removed, the positive trend becomes stronger for the remaining states.

Table 6.1 State characteristics and health and family welfare expenditure in India, around 1983

State	*Infant mortality rate (per 1,000) 1985*	*Per capita income (rupees) 1983–84*	*Plan per capita expenditure (rupees)*	*Nonplan per capita expenditure (rupees)*	*Total per capita expenditure (rupees)*
Andhra Pradesh	83	1,878	7	15	22
Assam	111	1,762	6	11	17
Bihar	106	1,174	5	8	13
Gujarat	98	2,795	9	19	29
Haryana	85	3,147	11	14	24
Himachal Pradesh	84	2,230	29	31	60
Jammu and Kashmir	85	1,820	9	32	41
Karnataka	69	1,957	8	18	26
Kerala	32	1,760	7	22	29
Madhya Pradesh	122	1,636	7	10	17
Maharashtra	68	3,032	10	18	28
Orissa	132	1,330	9	13	22
Rajasthan	108	1,881	8	15	24
Tamil Nadu	81	1,827	5	19	24
Uttar Pradesh	142	1,567	7	9	16
West Bengal	74	2,231	9	21	29

Note: This is a partial sample of states; those with incomplete data were excluded.
Source: Infant mortality: Stout 1989, table 2.4; income and population: Krister 1988, tables 1 and 2; expenditure: Rao, Kahn, and Prasad 1987, tables 4.1 and 4.10.

Figure 6.1 State per capita health and family welfare spending by per capita income, India, 1983
(rupees)

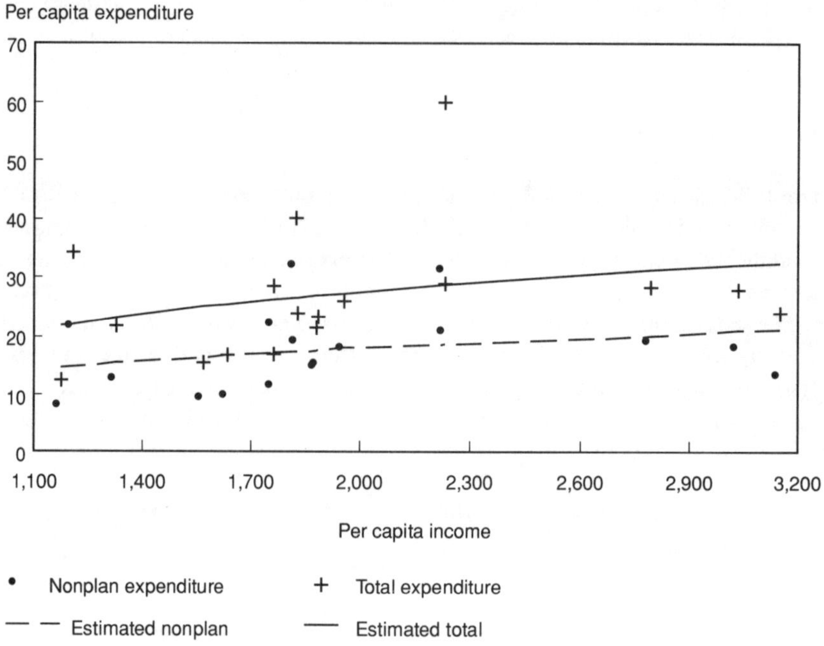

Source: Rao, Kahn, and Prasad 1987, and Krister 1988.

Figure 6.2 shows the relation between the infant mortality rate and per capita spending, which is negative. Higher infant mortality rates correspond to lower spending per capita. The low outlier for infant mortality at the bottom of the x-axis is the state of Kerala.[2]

Speeding up the progress in reducing infant mortality and slowing population growth, if public policies are to have any effect, presumably requires that these two relations be reversed—that public spending on health begin to favor poorer areas with worse health indicators. Health policy statements in India focus strongly on rural care, family welfare, and maternal and child health. Successful implementation of those policies, given the small role of central spending, would require that even state-level plan expenditure be higher where income is low and the infant mortality rate is high. But that is not the case, as figures 6.1 and 6.2 show, and a central problem of health policy in India is how to accomplish it.

Although infant mortality is negatively related to per capita income, neither of the figures controls for the other variable. If differences in income across states were controlled for, it might be expected that higher infant mortality rates would be associated with higher government spending. That is not the case: the negative relation between spending and infant mortality remains strong. When both variables enter a regression explaining nonplan per capita spending, the results show that a 1 percent increase in infant mortality is associated with a 0.5 percent drop in spending, while a 1 percent increase in per capita income is associated with a 0.5 percent increase in spending (the income coefficient is not significantly different from zero).[3]

If the same regression is run using just plan expenditure as the dependent variable, spending rises by 0.1 percent with a 1 percent increase in the infant mortality rate (this estimate is not significantly different from zero) but by 0.8 percent with a 1 percent increase in per capita income. Plan expenditure by states thus offsets slightly the negative relation between nonplan expenditure and infant mortality, but it reinforces the positive relation between nonplan expenditure and income.

The great unknown is whether central allocations offset or reinforce these state allocations, a crucial piece of information that has not been recovered from state budget documents. But the targeting criteria for the central budget are known. There is a set-aside of national allocations to the poorest states, and the remaining allocation is distributed on the basis of population (60 percent), per capita income below

Figure 6.2 State per capita health and family welfare spending by infant mortality rate, India, 1983

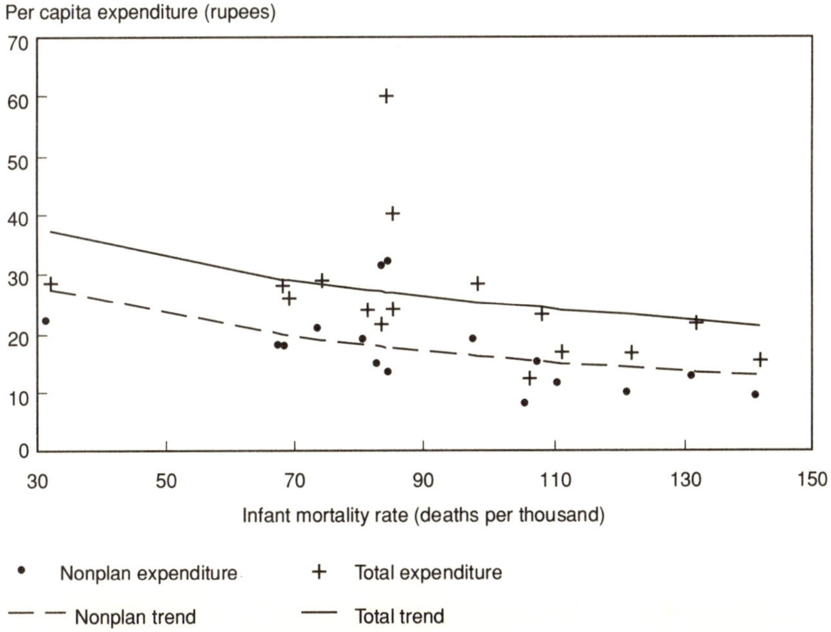

Source: Rao, Kahn, and Prasad 1987, and Stout 1989.

the national average (20 percent), state tax capacity (10 percent), and discretion (10 percent) (Indian Institute of Management 1987). Only the last category would allow targeting specifically by infant mortality or other criteria related to health and family welfare, so there is little chance that central funds could offset state allocations in that regard. There is more scope for central expenditure to offset the income effect than to allow targeting by health criteria.

In addition, central funds account for only 22 percent of plan expenditure and, as stated earlier, only 14 percent of total spending. Unless central funds are provided to states through means that affect how states spend their own money, the central government probably has little ability to influence states' health policy. In fact, central funds are allocated through block grants, often for programs paid for entirely from central funds. This approach probably skews state spending away from central government priorities except in programs that require a state contribution. Only data on actual patterns of spending by the central government could help unravel the total effect of these practices, but it seems unlikely that, under these allocation criteria, central funds could move the system strongly or rapidly in a new direction.

Targeting by program

Despite the lack of specific information on central budget allocations to states, examination of spending by programs can provide some information on spending priorities and how the central budget offsets or reinforces state patterns. Figure 6.3 and table 6.2 show the allocation of *state* spending (both plan and nonplan) in 1983 by program.[4] Approximately half of spending was allocated to secondary and tertiary curative services, including medical education. Spending on rural health services (including paramedic training and maternal and child care) and communicable disease control, two categories that on grounds of economic efficiency and health outcome should receive the greatest attention from governments, together accounted for about a fifth of spending. Family welfare, which in India is focused on sterilizations and not on more general health and population services, accounted for about 14 percent of state spending.

Figure 6.4 shows allocation of *central government* spending (both plan and nonplan) by the same programs. The central government appears to operate much like an international donor, concentrating primarily on capital expenditures for new programs, which account for nearly 40 percent of outlays. The family welfare program is nominally a centrally funded project, and it is clearly a high priority, consuming another 21 percent of the budget. Allocations to secondary and tertiary services, at 30 percent, absorb more than family welfare and about six times more than primary and rural care, another high-priority program.[5] Communicable disease control receives little central funding, which means that the central government has little capacity to offset regional imbalances in spending in that category.[6]

Because of the large role played by the state governments, central funds change

Figure 6.3 Distribution of state spending on health and family welfare, India, 1983
(percent)

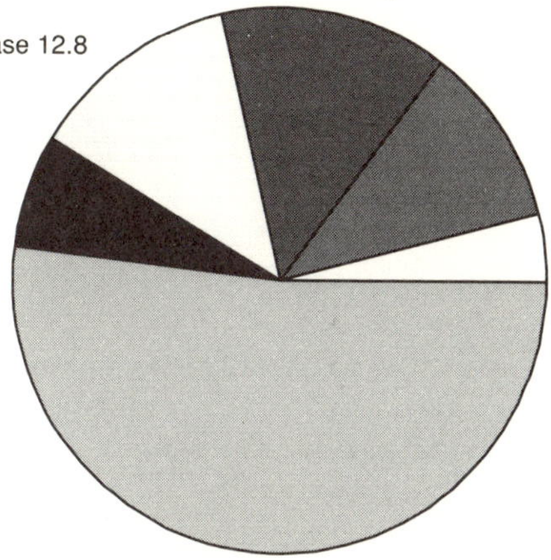

Source: Rao, Kahn, and Prasad 1987.

the targeting of programs only slightly, increasing the proportion allocated to family welfare and capital, and reducing the proportion spent on rural, communicable disease,[7] and secondary and tertiary activities. Overall, therefore, the distribution of aggregate central and state spending is close to that of state spending alone (see figure A.1 in the appendix).

Urban versus rural targeting

Evaluating public expenditure in health based on the relative concentration of spending in urban and rural areas is a much-abused method. Certain elements of a health system, usually the most expensive hospitals and training facilities, must be put in urban areas if they are to be utilized adequately and to employ specialized labor. In the more densely populated countries of Asia, locating these facilities in urban areas is less important than it is in the more sparsely populated countries of Africa and Latin America, but nowhere are hospitals put in the wilderness. Thus it is always easy to establish an urban bias for health spending, but some bias is inevitable and reflects economic necessity more than poor distribution of spending.

In India the urban bias in expenditure varies widely across states, but it is quite strong, and it is reinforced by an even stronger urban bias in central government spending. Overall, 41 percent of state spending goes to urban areas, and 19 percent

Table 6.2 Health and family welfare expenditure by program in India, 1983
(percent)

Program	*State spending*	*Central government spending*	*Total*
Administration	4.0	1.6	3.7
Secondary and tertiary			
Medical relief	39.3	6.1	34.7
Insurance	6.4	8.7	6.7
Medical education	6.1	15.2	7.4
Primary/rural			
Paramedical training	1.2	1.4	1.2
Rural health	4.5	0.7	4
Maternal and child health	1.0	2.9	1.3
Communicable disease	12.8	4.5	11.6
School health	0.1	0	0.1
Family planning	13.8	20.7	14.8
Other	8.1	11.2	8.5
Capital	2.7	26.9	6.1
Total	100	99.9	100
Rupees (thousands)	14,763,400	2,388,535	17,151,935
Percentage of total	86	14	100

Note: In chapter 4, an allocation of 71 percent to hospitals is used, which is based on other figures in the confusing source used for this table. From this table, hospitals would be calculated as consuming 64 percent of expenditure when family planning is removed and administration and capital are allocated to each program.
Source: Rao, Kahn, and Prasad 1987.

goes to rural areas, with 40 percent not allocated (table 6.3).[8] About 55 percent of central government expenditure is targeted to urban areas, and only about 1 percent to rural areas. Another 44 percent is common expenditures and cannot be allocated.

Rao, Kahn, and Prasad (1987) allocate common expenditures by population under the assumption that everyone benefits equally from them. Using this method produces results showing that 44 percent of expenditure in all of India was concentrated in urban areas in 1983, where 23.3 percent of the population lives. This implies that each urban resident receives 2.3 times the public health resources available to each rural resident. The last column in table 6.3 shows that the range of bias across states is 1.8 to 4.3, with a median value of 2.5. Figure A.2 in the appendix displays the share of population in rural areas by state, with the urban bias in expenditure on the right. Generally, about 80 percent of the states' population is rural, but city residents receive about twice the public health spending of their rural neighbors, and the bias tends to be higher in states with larger shares of their populations living in rural areas.

The assumption that all common expenditures are pure public goods that benefit everyone equally probably *minimizes* the measured urban bias because it is at least as likely that common expenditures are allocated in support of other expenditures. If

Figure 6.4 Distribution of central government allocation for health and family welfare, India, 1983
(percent)

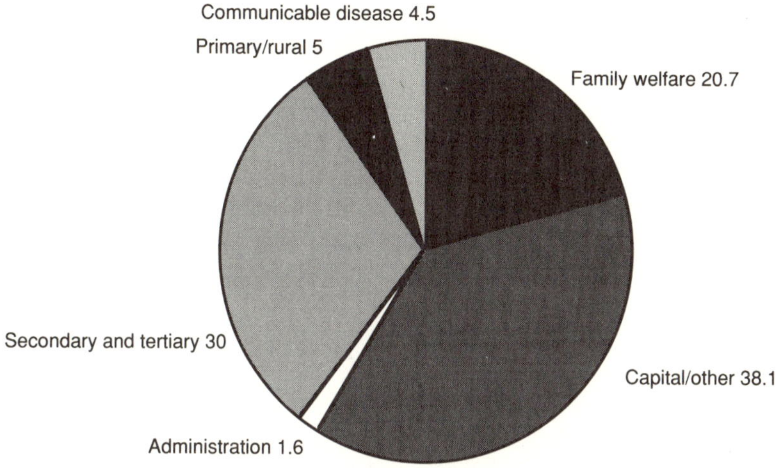

Source: Rao, Kahn, and Prasad 1987.

we assume that common expenditures have the same bias as those expenditures that can be allocated, 69 percent of state expenditures are devoted to urban areas, and the remainder, 31 percent, are targeted to rural areas. For the central government, 98 percent would be urban and only 2 percent rural. For total expenditures, 74 percent would be urban and 26 percent rural. The real urban allocation probably lies between the lower bound calculated by Rao, Kahn, and Prasad (1987) and the much higher percentage calculated by this method, but the ranking of states is not affected.

Summary

Nonplan health and family welfare spending (regular budget expenditure) by state governments in India is higher in wealthier states and lower in states with higher infant mortality rates. Although income and infant mortality are correlated, when income is controlled for, the negative relation between infant mortality and state spending is maintained. The relations between income and infant mortality rates and plan (special projects and capital) expenditure are similar, but weaker. Expenditure by the central government cannot be attributed to individual states using available data. However, given the relative size of the central allocation and the rules under which it is targeted, central spending may slightly offset the income effect but is unlikely to offset the infant mortality effect. If maternal and child health, rural health services, and control of infectious diseases are high priorities in government health policy, the policies have not yet been effectively translated into budget priorities.

Table 6.3 Distribution of health and family welfare expenditure between urban and rural areas in India, 1983
(percent)

State	*Urban*	*Rural*	*Common*	*Urban bias*
Andhra Pradesh	46.7	18.3	35.0	2.4
Assam	33.6	21.2	45.2	3.7
Bihar	23.5	28.4	48.1	2.4
Gujarat	43.0	13.2	43.8	1.8
Haryana	43.3	19.5	37.2	2.4
Himachal Pradesh	22.0	25.6	52.4	3.4
Jammu and Kashmir	52.5	18.1	29.4	2.8
Karnataka	44.1	17.5	38.4	1.9
Kerala	59.1	12.4	28.5	3.4
Madhya Pradesh	26.5	20.9	52.6	1.8
Maharashtra	47.7	7.8	44.5	1.8
Nagaland	39.0	17.1	43.9	3.0
Orissa	34.5	28.1	37.4	3.3
Rajasthan	44.6	17.4	38.0	2.5
Tamil Nadu	51.3	17.4	31.3	1.9
Tripura	43.4	18.3	38.3	4.3
Uttar Pradesh	36.1	18.4	45.5	2.5
West Bengal	48.1	16.0	35.9	2.2
States	41.1	18.6	40.3	2.6
Central government	55.4	0.9	43.7	
All India	44.0	15.1	40.9	2.3

Note: The calculation of urban bias is explained in the text.
Source: Rao, Kahn, and Prasad 1987.

Except for the amorphous capital spending category, the central government allocation by program generally parallels state allocations. The central government actually devotes a smaller proportion of its spending than states to communicable diseases, a category in which it might be expected to take a leadership role because of externalities across states and regions. Only in family welfare does the central government play a clearly positive role in allocating funds according to its objectives.[9] Common economic criteria that might guide the targeting of central funds, especially providing minimum levels of public goods, offsetting state-level differences in income, and targeting states with poor health statistics, do not appear to play an important role. Although the central government may direct capital spending to high-priority programs, that technique probably has a limited influence on the spending priorities of states. Targeting through capital spending is only one of several possible approaches and has serious limitations from a public finance standpoint.[10]

There is a strong urban bias to spending. A large percentage of spending in cities is fixed independent of the concentration of the population. However, the urban bias varies considerably across states, suggesting that considerable discretion is exercised in where and how funds are spent. The central government strongly boosts the state bias toward urban spending.

These biases can be corrected through a number of policy tools. Urban spending can be frozen at current levels, with additions to expenditure being targeted to rural areas until policymakers are satisfied that inequities have been redressed. If facilities and personnel must be located in urban areas, means can be found to extend their services to rural areas (through mobile clinics, satellite clinics, and ambulance services). User fees and insurance can be used to support urban programs that deliver private goods (such as curative services), with government funds allocated to programs that provide benefits extending beyond the individual (such as communicable disease control) and that lend themselves to geographical targeting. Central governments have many tools at their disposal to increase the effectiveness of their funds even when they control relatively small fractions of total spending. Matching grant programs and targeting of those programs by activity, geographical area, or political entity can result in changes in expenditure patterns that far exceed the actual amount of central funds allocated.

Government health and family welfare budgets will not grow rapidly enough to allow for significant, timely reallocations through new funds only. Retargeting expenditures will require reallocations of existing funds, and difficult choices for policymakers in India.

Public health expenditure in Indonesia

World Bank data can be used to show the distribution of health spending relative to provincial per capita income and infant mortality for Indonesia, in a manner similar to that used for India. Unlike the case in India, Indonesia's central government budget accounts for most public spending on health, 85 percent in 1985–86, with provincial governments accounting for 10 percent and districts accounting for 5 percent; and the central budget can be disaggregated by province.

Patterns of central and provincial/district allocations

Indonesia's public health spending, like India's, is positively correlated with provincial income (see appendix figure A.3).[11] The relation is particularly strong for provincial spending, with an income elasticity of 1.07. This result means that a 1 percent increase in provincial per capita income corresponds to a 1.07 percent increase in per capita health spending by provincial and district governments.[12] The pattern of central government spending on health reinforces this bias in provincial spending. The elasticity of such spending with respect to provincial income is 0.56, which is lower than the income elasticity of provincial spending, but nevertheless positive. The combined result is that average per capita income in the wealthiest province is 3.1 times higher than in the poorest province, provincial health spending is 3.0 times higher, and central government health spending is 2.2 times higher. Central government expenditure provides no offset to provincial inequalities.

A detailed analysis of budget channels used by the central government shows that the routine Central Ministry of Health budget most strongly reinforces provincial income patterns, with an income elasticity of 1.38. Even the income elasticity of the development budget for health centers is positive, at 0.41. Only the central government's salary grant to provinces (which pays salaries for centrally approved posts) has a slight negative relation to provincial income, with an elasticity of –0.10.

Differences in expenditure may not parallel differences in the quantity of services available in different provinces if, for example, not relatively expensive physicians, but relatively inexpensive paramedics, are targeted to provinces with high infant mortality. If this were the case, observing that spending is skewed to the higher-income provinces would not necessarily be an accurate representation of policy choices.

As might be expected, costly hospital beds are skewed toward the better-off provinces (figure 6.5), and the availability of beds is negatively linked to the infant mortality rate (figure 6.6). These relations are consistent with the earlier information on expenditure. The same patterns also hold in the distribution of paramedics working out of health centers (see appendix figures A.5 and A.6).[13] Primary health workers are apparently not targeted to the provinces with the poorest populations and worst health indicators. The distribution of health inputs and expenditures reflects the same skewed distribution of public resources in Indonesia.

Curative care spending and income distribution

To reach a more disaggregated level, information from a 1978 nationwide socioeconomic survey[14] can be combined with government health expenditure data to show the distribution of government subsidies to curative services across households, by income group. Two crucial assumptions underpin this analysis: use patterns across income groups are assumed to be approximately the same in 1986 as in 1978, and individuals are assumed to capture subsidies in direct proportion to the number of visits they make at each level of the system.[15]

As shown in table 6.4, 39 percent of government health spending cannot be attributed to specific activities and is labeled as "other." Consequently, only the budgets for hospitals and health centers are used in this analysis, with the training budget allocated to hospitals and health centers in proportion to their budget shares.[16] Thus the analysis concerns 59 percent of the total budget, basically the curative care budget, as it is accumulated in the last column of the table. Figure 6.7 displays the results of these manipulations and the allocation of government spending to clients according to their use patterns.

Government support of curative services is heavily biased toward the high-income group because of its relatively heavy use of hospitals. The poorest 40 percent of the

Figure 6.5 Relation between provinces' government hospital beds per capita and income per capita, Indonesia, 1985

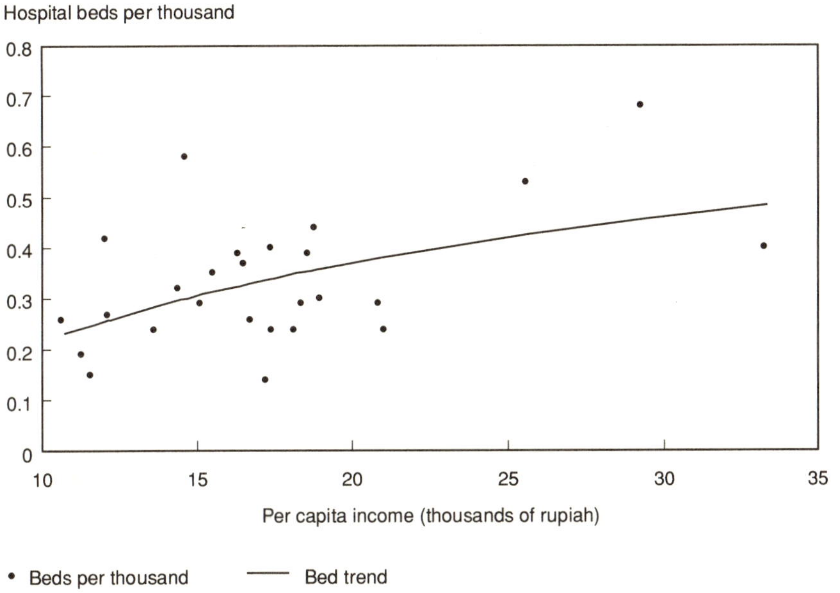

Source: World Bank data.

population captures about 17 percent of curative expenditure, the middle 30 percent captures about 31 percent, and the wealthiest 30 percent captures 52 percent. Although the poorest group captures a relatively larger share of expenditure in public health centers, it is more than offset by the large absolute size of hospital budgets and the extremely skewed distribution of hospital subsidies.

Summary

Indonesia's central government allocations appear, like India's, to be targeted to better-off provinces. But because funds from the central government play a larger role in Indonesia, it has a greater capacity to offset income differences across provinces and would have a large impact on spending priorities if it chose to target funds to poorer provinces or to provinces with higher infant mortality rates. This equity problem would be reduced even if funds were allocated to provinces purely on a per capita basis, which would at least remove the existing bias in favor of wealthier provinces.

Analysis of aggregate data at the provincial level indicates that spending patterns do not favor lower-income groups. But it captures only part of the story. As figure 6.7 shows, albeit with admittedly imprecise information, differences in government

Figure 6.6 Relation between provinces' government hospital beds per capita and infant mortality rate, Indonesia, 1985

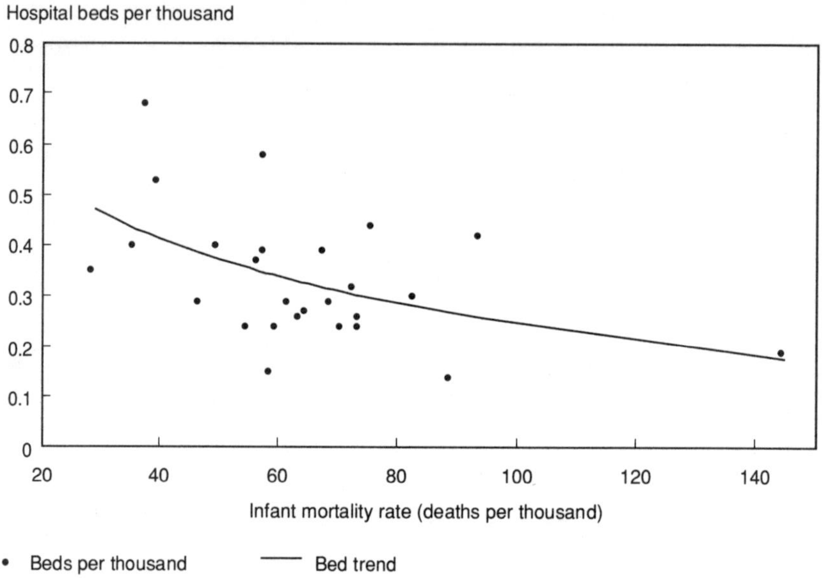

Source: World Bank data.

Table 6.4 Allocation of consolidated health budget in Indonesia, 1985–86

Item	*Total allocation (billions of rupiah)*	*Distribution (percent)*	*Totals used in analysis (billions of rupiah)*
Hospitals	208.0	33	225.2
Health centers	116.6	19	126.2
Communicable disease control	29.3	5	
Training	26.9	4	
Other	240.4	39	
Total	621.2	100	351.4

Source: World Bank data.

expenditures across income groups are much larger than those shown using aggregate provincial data. One reason is that customers' use patterns determine who benefits from curative care subsidies. Only those who use government facilities can receive a subsidy.[17] Curative expenditures by governments are highly skewed by use patterns toward higher-income groups in Indonesia. As with the provincial distribution of expenditures, distribution of government subsidies by head would result in a more equal distribution than is now the case.

Figure 6.7 Distribution of curative care subsidies by income group, Indonesia, 1985-86

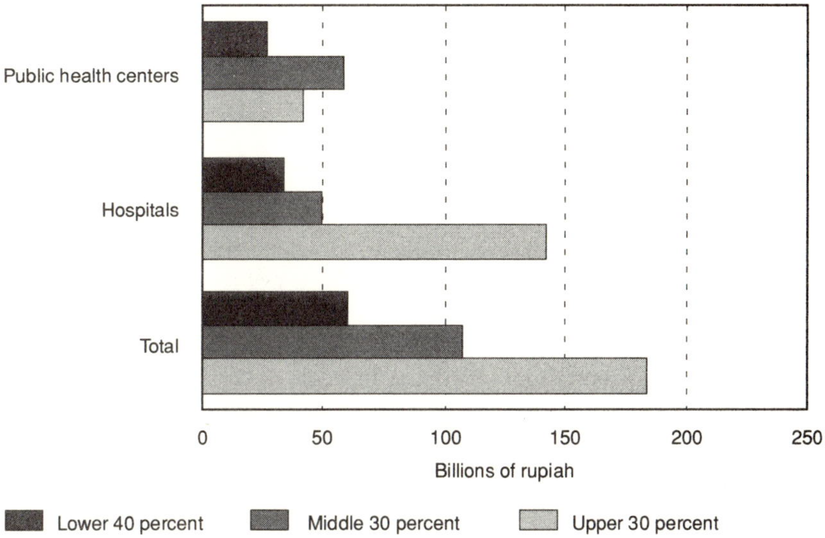

Source: World Bank data.

As was noted for India, public health activities (such as communicable disease control) are one of the government's main responsibilities. In Indonesia, about 90 percent of communicable disease expenditure comes from the central government, but it is small and falling (5 percent of spending in table 6.4). If all communicable disease spending were somehow captured by the poorest group (by geographical targeting, for example), its share of total spending in figure 6.7 would not rise to the next group's level. In fact, the communicable disease program was cut by 72 percent in 1987–88, effectively eliminating several important activities (such as tuberculosis and filariasis control) in order to maintain curative services.

Public health expenditure in Malaysia

Ministry of Health spending by state

An interstate analysis of expenditure is also possible for Malaysia, using data from 1983. As in India and Indonesia, a positive relation exists between Ministry of Health spending and state-level per capita GNP (see appendix figure A.7), while a negative relation exists between Ministry of Health spending and state-level infant mortality rates (see appendix figure A.8). Malaysia's infant mortality is, however, much lower than in the other two countries, with less variation across states, and there is a wider range of incomes across states (but with a higher overall average).

Closer inspection of those figures suggests that there is little dispersion in the data points except for one outlier in each case—the capital region (with high per capita income, a low infant mortality rate, and high spending). If the outlier is eliminated, the relation between spending and per capita income becomes flat (figure 6.8), and that between spending and the infant mortality rate becomes mildly positive (figure 6.9).[18]

In a regression analysis identical to the exercise for India and Malaysia, neither per capita GNP nor the infant mortality rate is statistically significant in explaining the distribution of expenditures, with or without the outlier. At worst, spending is not skewed toward the better-off states; at best, the Ministry of Health targets spending in such a way as to eliminate the income effect. Similarly, its spending is at least not diverted away from states with high infant mortality rates. The apparently equal per capita spending across states shown in figure 6.8 is redistributive in the sense that it represents 2.6 percent of per capita GNP in the poorest state but only 0.8 percent in the richest state.

Figure 6.8 Ministry of Health spending and per capita GNP by state, Malaysia, 1983
(outlier removed; Malaysian dollars)

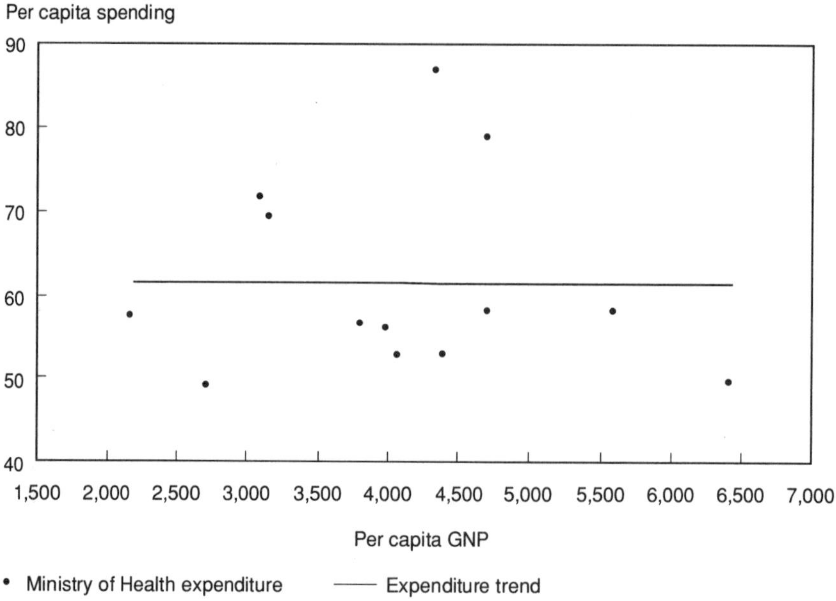

Source: Westinghouse Health Systems and Government of Malaysia 1985.

Figure 6.9 Ministry of Health spending and infant mortality rate by state, Malaysia, 1983 *(outlier removed)*

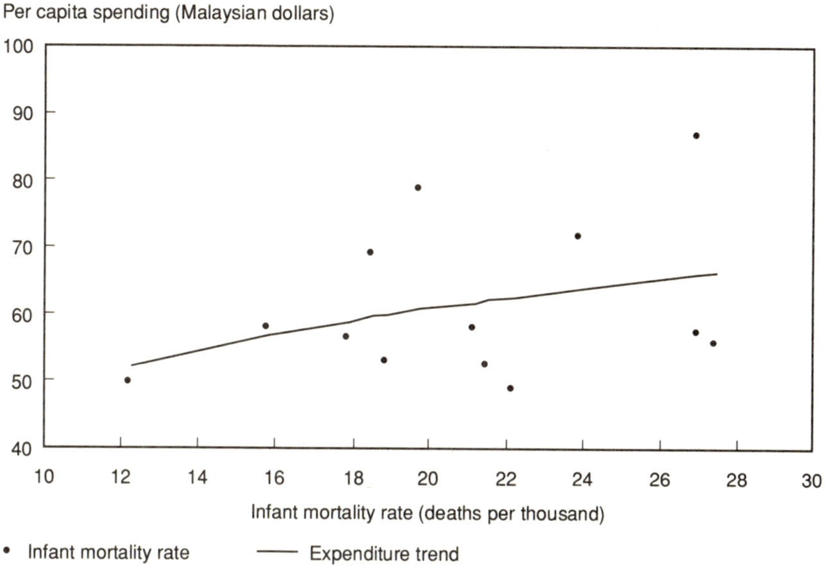

Source: Westinghouse Health Systems and Government of Malaysia 1985.

Detailed analysis of the distribution of public expenditures

Meerman's rigorous analysis (1979) of the distributive impact of government health care spending for Malaysia for the mid-1970s provides a dated but complete picture of subsidy patterns that reinforces this aggregate picture. The analysis is old and well known, so only the principal results are presented here.

Figure 6.10 shows the distribution of public subsidies by type of curative institution as well as for public health activities. For the sake of clarity, only three of the five income quintiles are shown. For curative services, subsidies are allocated to quintiles according to their use patterns as they were revealed in a national survey designed for the purpose. For public health activities, subsidies are assumed to be distributed equally on a per capita basis, a reasonable assumption for public goods.[19]

The results are plain to see and easy to understand. Hospital inpatient subsidies have no clear pattern across income groups, presumably because they are captured by virtue of catastrophic, low-probability illnesses that are unrelated to income. Because inpatient services are costly, the absolute size of that untargeted subsidy dwarfs subsidies available through other parts of the system and contributes to a total subsidy pattern similar to that for inpatients.

Figure 6.10 Government health expenditure per capita by type of program or service and by income group, Malaysia, 1973

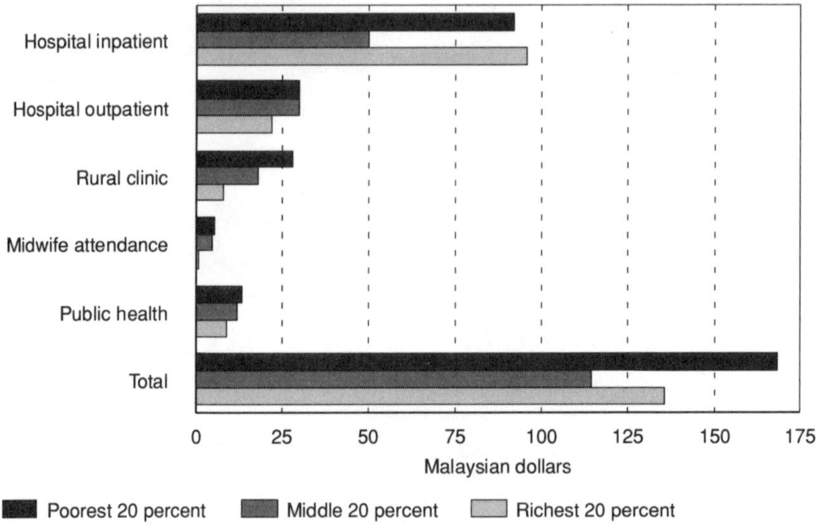

Source: Meerman 1979.

Parts of the system are redistributive. Spending on hospital outpatient services slightly favors the poor, and rural clinic services and midwifery attendance for births are targeted to the poorer quintiles. Public health expenditures are mildly progressive because poorer households are larger, and thus contain more beneficiaries of the equal per capita subsidy. Figure 6.11 shows how the full budget for each program is captured by the five income quintiles (from poorest on the left to richest on the right). The results reinforce these observations. The poorest 20 percent captures significantly more than 20 percent of the subsidy only from rural clinics and midwives. In carefully targeted programs a reasonable goal might be for the poorest 40 percent to capture 75 percent or more of public subsidies, which is far from the case here.

One of the main reasons for the favorable distribution of public spending for hospital outpatient and rural clinic services is that all groups have about the same number of visits per year (the mean is 12.42 per household),[20] but use of private sector services increases monotonically from an average of 1.36 visits per year for the poorest group to 6.72 visits per year for the richest group. Thus wealthier households self-select themselves out of the public sector even though they could use it for the same price as the poor. Other evidence not discussed here indicates that public expenditures are also well targeted to residents of rural areas, where more of the poorer households are located.

Figure 6.11 Spending for government health programs by household income quintile, Malaysia, 1973

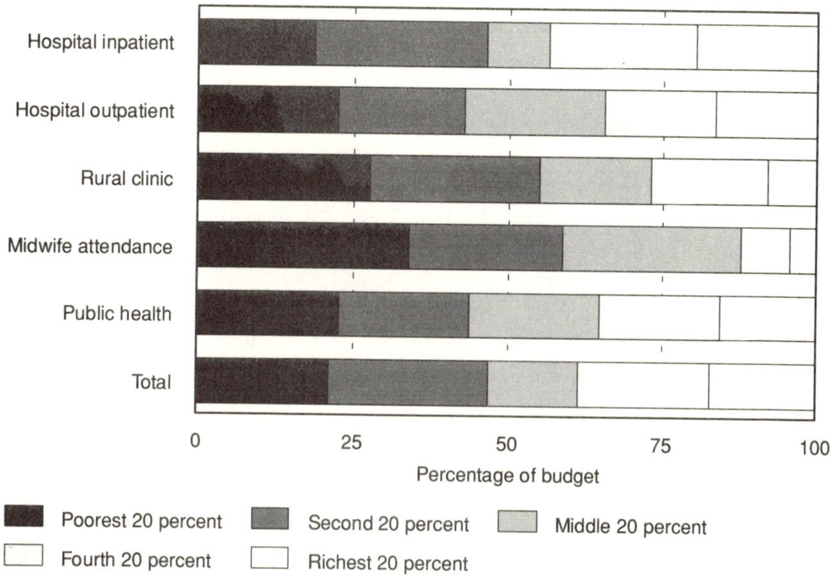

Source: Meerman 1979.

Summary

The statistics for Malaysia show that it is possible to target subsidies to states that have greater need because of low incomes, high infant mortality, or both. Malaysia does not redistribute health spending to such a degree that it creates a negative relation between spending and provincial income or a positive relation between spending and infant mortality in a regression analysis, but both are at least rendered neutral.

Although total subsidies are not strongly redistributive across households, subsidies are targeted to some important but relatively inexpensive services that benefit the poor disproportionately (these include rural clinics, midwives, and public health spending). The more detailed analysis provides the first indication that interactions between the public and private sectors can help to target public subsidies better if the higher-income groups tend to use the private sector. User fees, means tests, and insurance coverage for higher-income households would allow the government to target its health subsidies even more narrowly, especially for hospital inpatient and outpatient services.

Targeting public expenditure in Papua New Guinea

Figure 6.12 shows the trend across 17 of 19 rural provinces in spending on hospital and rural services by governments and missions in Papua New Guinea. Most government spending comes directly or indirectly from the central government. The government pays for basically the same personnel and supplies in mission clinics that it provides to government clinics, although the missions are free to add to these contributions using their own resources.[21] Government hospital spending per capita is positively related to provincial income, and the trend is steep for the poorest provinces. Spending on rural government health services is also positively related to income, but less so than hospital spending. Total spending on rural services, which adds subsidies through missions to the government's direct services, is nearly constant across income levels, so the mission subsidy tends to compensate for lower direct government spending in the poorer provinces. Because there is less spending on hospitals per capita than on rural services, the greater equality across provinces in expenditure targeted to rural areas represents a real offset to the more skewed hospital spending.

Figure 6.13 shows the relation between infant mortality in 1980 and spending in 1986. Using a lagged value for spending is actually preferable to concurrent observations on spending and infant mortality because it allows for possible increases in spending by policymakers reacting to earlier information on infant mortality. The

Figure 6.12 Health spending and per capita income by province, Papua New Guinea, 1986 *(kina)*

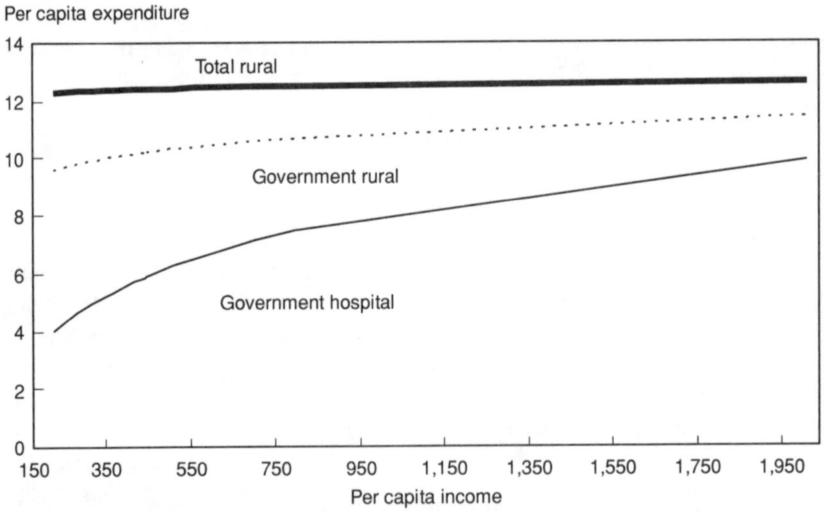

Source: Thomason and Newbrander 1988, and World Bank data.

Figure 6.13 Health spending and infant mortality rate by province, Papua New Guinea, 1986

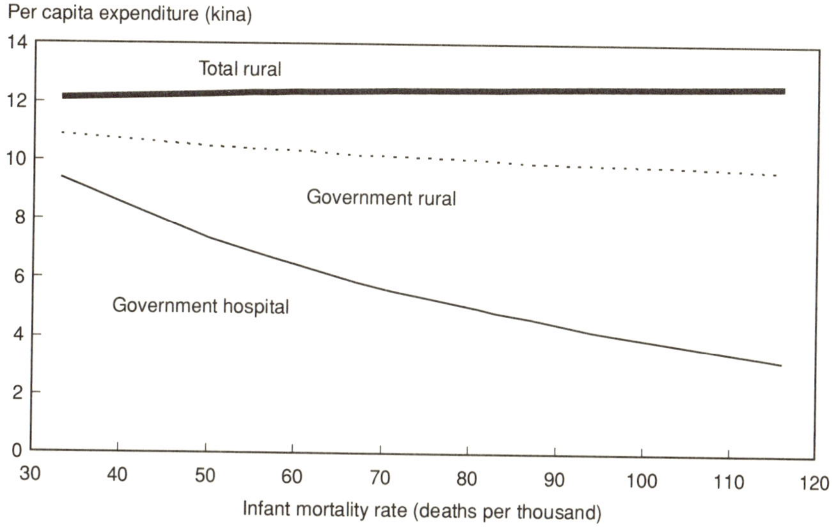

Source: Thomason and Newbrander 1988, and World Bank data.

results are similar to those for income. Hospital spending drops off steeply as the infant mortality rate rises; rural spending by the government ameliorates this pattern; and subsidies through missions push total rural spending toward a faintly positive relation with infant mortality.

In a regression similar to those run earlier, with the logs of per capita income and infant mortality explaining the log of expenditure, the only significant relation is a negative one between infant mortality and hospital expenditure (with income controlled). All other specifications are insignificant, indicating no systematic relation between income or infant mortality and spending on health care other than on hospitals.

The result suggests that Papua New Guinea has eliminated the positive effect of income on rural health expenditure that was detected in several other countries, but it has not reversed it. It has also eliminated the bias against areas with high infant mortality in its spending on rural services, but it has not reversed it. In both cases, subsidies through missions on rural services improve targeting to the poorer provinces and to those with higher infant mortality.[22] The entire picture would be much more inequitable if the National Capital District could be included in the analysis, because it has by far the highest per capita income and the lowest infant mortality rate, and it accounts for about half of all government health spending. Moreover, it is isolated from other parts of the country, so expenditures there are not readily accessible to most of the 85 percent of the population living in rural areas. Yet to eliminate this subsidy pattern would require either eliminating the country's only tertiary care facility or dramatically increasing spending outside the capital in a country that already spends 10 percent of its public budget on health.

Recurrent health expenditure in Bangladesh

In Bangladesh, as in India, government spending is reported in two budgets. The capital and recurrent costs of new programs are funded through the development budget, and recurring costs of existing programs are funded through the revenue budget. About half the expenditures for clinics and most expenditures for field operations are in the development budget, a large share of which is financed by external donors. In contrast, most expenditures for hospitals, Upazila Health Complexes (small hospitals), and about half the Union Health and Family Welfare Centers (rural clinics) come from the revenue budget, which is financed entirely from domestic funds. The discussion in this section relates only to health expenditures in the revenue budget.

Successful retargeting to rural areas

The government of Bangladesh spent about $1.12 per capita on health in 1987, about half of it through the revenue budget. The overall revenue budget increased steeply over the last decade in nominal terms (appendix figure A.9). Although health spending also increased, in real terms, the increase has been uneven. For several years in the 1980s health spending fell as a percentage of the total budget, but by 1988 it accounted for 5.2 percent of the total, compared with 4.1 percent in 1978. In real terms, spending declined by up to 20 percent of the 1978 level, although it recovered in the last two years and now slightly exceeds real spending in 1978. Consequently, the apparent increases in revenue budget expenditure correspond to almost a flat trend in real terms.

Figure 6.14 shows just the health part of the budget, with a clearer representation of urban and rural spending on curative services. Urban and rural hospitals and clinics account for almost all revenue budget spending, either directly or indirectly. The unallocated funds in figure 6.14 are spent largely in support of hospitals and clinics. The expansion of rural hospitals and clinics resulted, for the first time in 1983, in larger budget allocations for rural curative services than for urban services in this country where 88 percent of the population is rural. Because the total budget did not increase substantially in real terms, this reallocation has meant a real decline in resources for urban facilities, an exceptional achievement in the retargeting of curative expenditures.

The reallocation of spending on curative services is corroborated by information on health inputs. Between 1976 and 1985, the number of Upazila Health Complexes (31-bed rural hospitals serving about 225,000 people each) rose from 150 units with

Figure 6.14 Trends in hospital and clinic revenue spending, Bangladesh, 1978-88

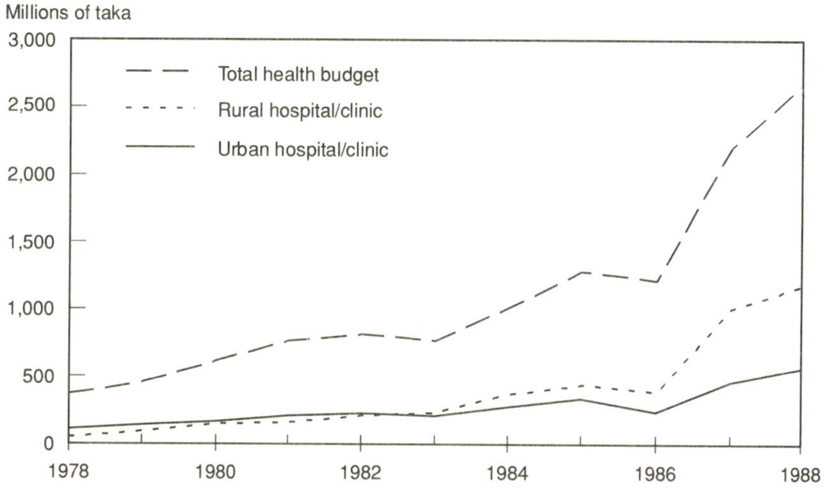

Source: IBA 1988.

900 beds to 341 units with 6,820 beds (BIDS 1988). The country also added about 1,000 Union Health and Family Welfare Centers, which are outpatient facilities designed to serve about 25,000 people each. It also trained and hired more than 10,000 field-workers.

Unexpected consequences of retargeting

Because the change was accomplished within a fixed budget, the improved targeting has probably resulted in a somewhat more costly but lower-quality curative system. Figure 6.15 shows revenue budget allocations per patient at each level of the curative system[23] on the left, with bed occupancy rates on the right. Although the case mix and complexity of services offered at the higher-level institutions would undoubtedly favor higher costs, spending per patient is astoundingly low. At an exchange rate of 32.27 taka to the dollar, the costs in the graph range from $3.07 in the most expensive institution to $0.59 in the least expensive. The top institutions are extremely efficient, or they provide a low level of care, or their patients provide many of the inputs themselves. All three hypotheses probably contain some truth.

The difference in unit costs is also partially due to differences in utilization. A typical Upazila Health Complex has an annual budget that is about half that of a 100-bed district hospital, but it treats less than half the number of outpatients, and half its beds are usually empty. Yet increasing the utilization of these lower-level facilities may raise unit costs considerably above current levels. At this time, most have

Figure 6.15 Hospital and clinic unit costs and utilization rates, Bangladesh, 1978-88

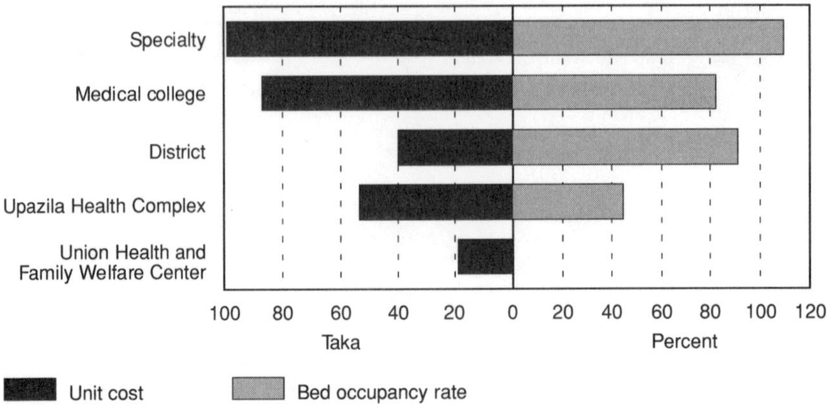

Source: IBA 1988.

inadequate staff and no blood bank, x-ray machine, or basic laboratory equipment. Even if utilization rises faster than costs (resulting in lower unit costs), the total costs of the facilities would rise against a stagnant health budget. The prognosis for these facilities is not good without new sources of revenue.

Thus the Bangladesh experience presents a conundrum. The country has succeeded in shifting recurrent curative care spending toward rural hospitals and clinics, but this has been accomplished by taking resources out of more centralized and apparently more efficient higher-level facilities, widening access to the system but probably not increasing either the quantity or the quality of services delivered. This hypothesis is supported by the fact that inpatient visits to higher-level public facilities have at best stayed constant since 1983, and outpatient visits have declined (Griffin 1989)—an extraordinary outcome in a country with virtually no private hospitals and a population that is growing by about 3 million a year.

Survey evidence on rural targeting by individuals

A related question is how far the retargeting of hospital and clinic expenditure in a poor country such as Bangladesh really moves it toward its health policy goals. As in many countries, at the top of the list of goals for Bangladesh is a reduction in the infant mortality rate, an increase in life expectancy, and a reduction in fertility, all of which presumably require that a substantial portion of expenditure be targeted to women and children.

A set of household and facility surveys conducted in Bangladesh in 1987 provides information on how curative care spending through rural facilities is distributed relative to these health needs. In the household survey, 2,400 rural and 500 urban households were visited. Behavior in the two samples was different, but the focus here is on the rural sample (BIDS 1988). All health facilities serving the surveyed households were also visited (IBA 1988).

In each facility samples of outpatients and inpatients were interviewed on the day of the field interviewer's visit. In rural areas the facilities visited were primarily the Upazila Health Complex and the Union Health and Family Welfare Center; only results from these visits will be reported here.[24] Of 621 rural patients visiting the government clinics, only 7 percent were children 5 years old or younger. About 56 percent of the patients were between the ages of 16 and 40. Females accounted for only 36 percent of the patients. Thus the dispersion of curative services into rural areas in the manner chosen by the government does not necessarily lead to a distribution of subsidies among patients that is consistent with its stated policies, although it did increase the share of government spending going to rural areas. If the facility sample is somewhat representative of actual patterns, it suggests that a heavily male-biased group age 16–40 is the main group capturing the subsidies. Fewer than 5 percent of the visits had to do with family planning, obstetrical care, or prenatal care.

Results from the household survey—which capture reported use of any types of health care service—do not correspond closely to these patterns of use at government facilities, possibly because of the nonrandom selection of respondents in the facility survey. Figure 6.16 shows the distribution of consumption by type of health service in various age groups. For no age group does the government provide more than 14 percent of the services sought, but the private sector provides over 50 percent for all groups. According to this information, the facility survey should have found that 27 percent of the government patients were under age 5, 21 percent were age 5–14, 39 percent were age 15–49, and 13 percent were over age 50, numbers that are quite different than those the sample actually collected. Interestingly, the same distribution of patients would be calculated for private and traditional practitioners as well, based on the data underlying figure 6.16. In other words, use patterns at government clinics do not appear to be particularly successful in reaching target population groups—young children, and females of childbearing ages.

Taken together, the data suggest that the government's expenditures through its clinic- and hospital-based rural system are not targeted differently than private expenditures. Furthermore, the government provides such a small percentage of these services relative to what rural people actually consume that it is difficult to detect how it could make a difference. This is affirmed by figure 6.17 and appendix figure A.11, which show use patterns by the education of the household head and operational landholdings. The government provides a slightly larger share of services used by the least educated and poorest group, but the impact is almost negligible. (For figure 6.17, the group with no education accounts for 68 percent of the sample of sick people; for figure A.11, the group with less than 0.5 acres accounts for 64 percent of the sample.) Looked at from the opposite angle, free government services are also leaking to small groups of the educated and landed elite.

Figure 6.16 Type of health care used by ill patients on day of survey, by age group, rural Bangladesh, 1987

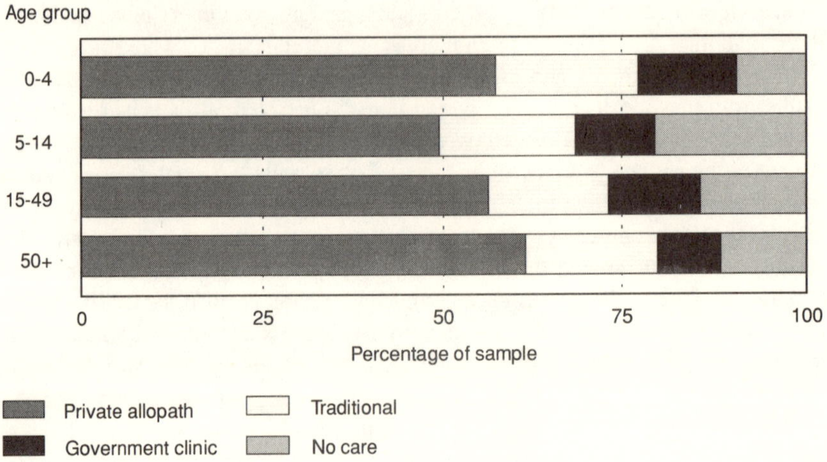

Source: BIDS 1988.

Figure 6.17 Type of health care used, by education of household head, Bangladesh, 1987

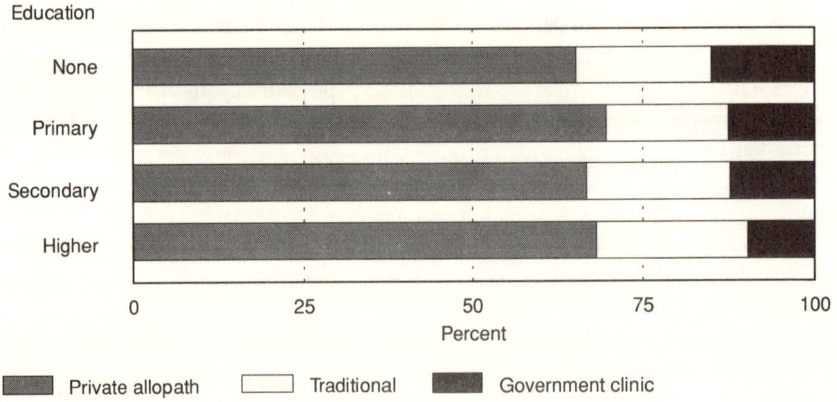

Source: BIDS 1988.

Finally, the household sample contains complete information on demand patterns related to current pregnancies and pregnancies during the previous year. Only 16 percent of the currently pregnant rural women received any kind of prenatal care. Of 677 rural women who either were currently pregnant or had given birth during the previous year, 99 percent either planned to or did deliver at home with a relative or an ordinary dai (traditional midwife) in attendance. Fewer than 10 percent of the children age 0–4 had any immunization. For all practical purposes, there is little modern medical attention before birth, none at birth, and almost none after birth.

In the rural sample, children under age 5 accounted for 15 percent of the population but 45 percent of the deaths. About half those deaths were attributed by respondents to diarrhea or diseases that immunization can prevent. In a typical village of 2,000 people, the investigators from the Bangladesh Institute of Development Studies calculated that one or two mothers and 15 children under age 5 would die each year.

Summary

Bangladesh's experience shows how complex a policy issue targeting can be. While the country has succeeded in targeting a greater proportion of its curative spending to rural areas, the result is a more dispersed system operating with almost the same resources that were devoted to a much smaller system 10 years ago. Moreover, the simple extension of clinics and hospitals into rural areas has created public expenditure and subsidy patterns that tend to mimic existing private expenditure patterns. Thus, the allocation of government spending does not compensate for deficiencies in the pattern of private expenditures, which are not directed toward health care during and after pregnancy. The recurrent budget simply does not reach groups that the government's own health policy would indicate should be targeted. As a result, the clear shift in curative care subsidies to the countryside in the last decade, while laudable, has apparently not directed subsidies to high-priority individuals (mainly women of childbearing age and their children) in any systematic way.[25]

Conclusion

Government provision of public health goods—control of infectious diseases, safe drinking water, sewerage facilities, regulation of air and water pollution, and so on—has redistributive effects, albeit not well quantified, since the poor tend to suffer most when public investments in these goods are inadequate. By definition, public goods are untargeted, but their redistributive effects can be enhanced if investments are directed specifically to impoverished areas and disadvantaged population groups. In all countries, the aggregate pattern of distribution depends on the division of funding responsibility between central and lower levels of government, particularly the relative sizes of their budgets, and the extent to which the spending patterns in one budget are reinforced or offset by those in the other.

The foregoing discussion documents the outcomes in India, Indonesia, Malaysia, Papua New Guinea, and Bangladesh. India is the only country in this group in which state government resources make up the bulk of total public health resources (86 percent). Neither central nor state government spending is particularly targeted toward poor areas or population groups. Urban residents, for example, capture nearly 2.5 times as much of the total public health expenditure as their population share, and spending levels are negatively related to infant mortality rates (an indicator of general health conditions in the locality), contrary to what might be expected on grounds of equity, or even health.

In the other countries, central government spending is the main determinant of patterns of allocation. Bangladesh has the unusual record of having retargeted spending toward rural areas in the last decade, but because overall spending is so low the result has been a dilution of the quality of government health services, and a failure to channel subsidies toward lower-income groups. It is widely believed that usage rates at public rural clinics have dropped as people have sought nongovernment services because of the low quality and poor functioning of public facilities. A fundamental flaw in the retargeting effort appears to lie in the failure to reorient spending away from curative toward primary health services and public health activities.

In Indonesia and Papua New Guinea, central government spending also benefits better-off groups. In Papua New Guinea, for example, the National Capital District absorbs a disproportionate share of the sector's total resources even though it has the lowest rate of infant mortality. Outside the District, allocations of health spending through government facilities continue to favor better-off areas, but the bias is offset almost completely by subsidies through religious missions, which apparently tend to be located in poorer areas. The experience testifies to a potentially powerful role for charitable organizations as conduits of public resources to the rural poor.

Malaysia stands alone in contrast to the other countries in the sample for which the geographical distribution of expenditures could be determined: its lowest-income groups appear to capture a fair share of total public subsidies for health, and spending across localities shows a flat rather than a positive link to incomes. The Malaysian experience suggests that it is possible to avoid biases against the poorest areas and those with the worst health indicators in the allocation of public health resources if other supporting strategies, including user fees, means tests, and insurance coverage, are in place to encourage higher-income groups to self-select against using government services.

The language of this chapter has been characterized by negatives. The most redistributive result that has been uncovered, in Malaysia, is characterized above as suggesting "that it is possible to avoid biases against the poorest areas and those with the worst health indicators." If governments were truly in the business of offsetting income and health inequalities, and of supplementing private expenditure with public health inputs (which is certainly the rhetoric), observed public expenditure patterns would be reversed. The attractive finding in this chapter is that existing spending patterns are so far from what might be expected that most governments have extraordinary opportunities to improve the health of their citizens simply by improving the targeting of existing public expenditure.

Notes

1. Not all the data are for the same year, and not all Indian states are represented. The infant mortality rate is for 1984–85; per capita income is for 1983–84; spending is for 1982–83; population figures used to calculate per capita spending are for 1981. No data could be assembled for Punjab and Manipur, and other states have missing cells. Any states with missing data were not used in the regression analysis.

2. The equation is log(per capita nonplan expenditure) = 1.7 – 0.53*log(IMR) + 0.46*log(per capita income). The coefficient on infant mortality is statistically significant with a t-ratio of 2.09; the coefficient on per capita income is not statistically significant at commonly accepted levels, with a t-ratio of 1.39. The regression as a whole is significant at the 0.97 level, with an R-square of 0.41.

3. Although this regression implies a causal relation between the infant mortality rate and income, on one hand, and spending, on the other, certainly causation goes both ways. The intention in performing this analysis is to show whether there is a relation. Seeing a high infant mortality rate, a policymaker might spend more in the expectation that the infant mortality rate would then fall. If policymakers behaved that way, we would observe a positive relation between infant mortality and spending. Because a negative relation is observed, this decision pattern is not verified. If infant mortality were on the left and expenditures were on the right, the relation would still be negative, indicating that spending less on health and family welfare results in higher infant mortality, even when controlling for income. At the level of precision possible with this small sample and the data, all that matters is that there is a negative relation. The data imply in one specification that to reduce the infant mortality rate, more will have to be spent; the other specification shows that in fact less is spent where infant mortality is worse.

4. A more detailed list of allocations is shown in table 6.2, which makes clear how the composite categories shown in the figures were created.

5. These statements do not take into account capital expenditure, which is equivalent to assuming that capital expenditure is allocated similarly to recurrent expenditure across programs.

6. Through migration and travel across state boundaries, citizens from states with relatively low allocations for communicable disease control may carry diseases to other states. Their citizens may also use subsidized health facilities in other states, becoming a burden on other government entities because of their own state's spending patterns. The failure of one state to spend adequately on communicable disease control may also reduce the effectiveness of efforts in neighboring states (for example, mosquitos and rivers cross state boundaries). Thus it would be efficient for the central government to enforce minimum acceptable disease control efforts across states and to ensure that adequate funding is available, quite apart from equally important equity considerations.

7. The malaria eradication program accounts for 85 percent of spending on communicable diseases. The expanded immunization program has been put under the primary/rural category.

8. Rao, Kahn, and Prasad (1987) use these classifications—urban: medical relief, excluding primary health care and rural dispensaries, medical education, urban services; rural: primary health care, rural services, dai training, village health guide training; common: administration, paramedical training, capital (except for primary health care, which is under rural), maternal and child health care and expanded immunization programs, mass education, family welfare compensation, research, public health.

9. It is going too far, however, to say that the central government supplements state spending on family planning, because its allocation of funds through block grants may displace state spending that would otherwise take place.

10. One of the main limitations is that it is rational for a government unit to accept almost any capital subsidy. That does not obligate the receiving entity to fund the recurrent costs necessary to make the program work.

11. As in India, the link between infant mortality and health spending (provincial and central) is downward sloping (see appendix figure A.4), although the relationship is not statistically significant when income is held constant.

12. The equation for this estimate is the following: log(provincial per capita health spending) = –3.39 + 1.07*log(provincial per capita household expenditure) –0.14*log (provincial infant mortality rate). Per capita household expenditure has a t-statistic of 2.8, which is highly significant. The infant mortality rate has a t-statistic of 0.42, which is not statistically significant. The regression as a whole is significant at above the 99 percent level, with an R-square of 0.39.

13. Paramedics working in hospitals are not included.

14. This is the SUSENAS survey; see Chernichovsky and Meesook (1986) for a description of it and an analysis of the health data.

15. This assumption is admittedly only an approximation, but at the aggregative level of the analysis pursued here, the main interest is in the relative magnitude of expenditures across groups, not the precise numbers. With the reduction of poverty in Indonesia during this period, it is likely that use rates among the poor have increased, and—at best—the bias in favor of richer groups may have declined somewhat. On the other hand, the use of medical services is highly income elastic, so—at worst—all groups may use more care, but the rich may have expanded their use even faster than the poor.

16. The health center budget category may be underreported by 60 percent or more, but its absolute size is not as important as the distribution for this section.

17. This statement is not entirely correct. The presence of government hospitals and health clinics reduces the risk of death—say, from an accident—even for those who do not use the services in a given year. Thus there is an insurance benefit for users and nonusers alike. It seems plausible that the insurance benefit should be allocated in proportion to use by each income class. Unless another rule is used, this insurance element would consequently not affect the distribution shown in figure 6.7, and it is probably quite small.

18. If the outliers are removed from the graphs for India and Indonesia, in contrast, the observed trends are either strengthened or not changed.

19. Because public health activities are often specific to geographic regions, they could be allocated more precisely if the necessary detail were available on spending patterns.

20. Equal numbers of visits mean fewer visits per capita for poorer households, however.

21. Several caveats are in order. The figure does not include spending in Port Moresby, the wealthiest area of the country, where national hospital services are located. Thus the discussion is really about rural spending. All but one of the provinces have per capita incomes below 800 kina (where the relations are strongest), but the outlier (at 1,973 kina) is included because it does not affect the relation. To limit the clutter the data points are not shown in these graphs; considerable variability around the trends is masked as a consequence. The solid line labeled "government hospital" shows hospital spending across provinces. The dotted "government rural" line is not additive and shows that in all provinces rural clinic and aid post spending is higher than hospital spending. The thick "total rural" line adds mission subsidies to the "government rural" line.

22. But of course the government may have lower direct spending in those provinces because subsidies through the missions there substitute for direct public service delivery.

23. This is calculated by dividing the total recurring expenditure in 1986–87 by the total number of patients, including both inpatients and outpatients. It does not include medicines and supplies or training and central administrative costs, but those costs are unlikely to change significantly the picture of relative costs that emerges from the graph.

24. The choice of respondents depends partly on the interviewer's preference, so the data may be biased by nonrandom sampling.

25. Readers familiar with Bangladesh might argue that the focus on the revenue budget in this presentation provides an inaccurate picture of the system (especially in regard to mothers and children) because most family welfare, field staff, mother and child health, and half of Union Health and Family Welfare Clinic expenditures are in the development budget. But that contention is probably wrong. The survey data are insensitive to which budget pays for the government clinics, so that is not an issue. Family welfare expenditures and family welfare workers are designed to promote sterilizations and intrauterine devices and, to a lesser extent, to provide other contraceptives. They have virtually no responsibilities in health. Field-workers with health responsibilities are male, so they are unlikely to have any impact on obstetrical or child care practices.

7

Conclusion

Health conditions

Progress in improving health and reducing population growth rates in Asia has been strong over the last 20 years, although the experience there has not been demonstrably different from that in other developing regions. There are persistent, large differences in performance among countries. For the sample of Asian countries, average female life expectancy at birth is about 62 years, but very few countries lie near the mean (table 7.1). Rather, there are three groups: five countries with female life expectancies below 60, three countries at about the mean, and four countries with female life expectancies at about 70 years. Several characteristics of these countries stand out.

• *Income versus policy.* While the poorer countries tend to be in the group with the lowest life expectancy, that is not uniformly the case. China and Sri Lanka are low-income countries that enjoy exceptional health indicators. Perhaps the potential effect of policies on health outcomes is best demonstrated by a hypothetical example. If it is assumed for the moment that countries can increase life expectancy only by increasing per capita GNP, a country such as Bangladesh could expect to increase female life expectancy by five to eight years if it doubled per capita income over the next decade. That would mean life expectancy for women of about 56 years in the year 2000 and per capita income of about $320. To achieve this improvement in life expectancy through income growth only would require real growth in GNP per capita of about 7 percent a year, an annual growth rate about 23 times higher than that typical for Bangladesh over the past 20 years.

In contrast, the experiences of China, India, Myanmar, and Sri Lanka show that policy decisions made in the social sectors could result in improvement in female life expectancy in Bangladesh of between 7 and 20 years by the year 2000 even without rapid income growth. Although income should not be discounted as a determinant of improvements in health, policy choices in the health sector can and do offset constraints imposed by low incomes. Although there is little evidence measuring the unique

Table 7.1 Female and male life expectancies and infant mortality rates, by female life expectancy group, in selected Asian countries, 1986

Female life expectancy and country	*Life expectancy*		*Infant mortality rate (per 1,000)*
	Female	*Male*	
Below 60 years			
Nepal	47	48	130
Bangladesh	50	51	121
Papua New Guinea	54	51	64
India	56	57	86
Indonesia	58	55	87
Between 60 and 66 years, inclusive			
Myanmar	61	58	64
Philippines	65	62	46
Thailand	66	62	41
Over 66 years			
China	70	68	34
Malaysia	71	67	27
Sri Lanka	72	68	29
Korea	73	66	25

Source: Appendix table A.2.

effect of health policies on health outcomes, one cannot come away from this study without realizing that countries have made divergent choices in levels and allocation of support for the health sector, and that these different choices lead to differences in health outcomes that begin to show up over time.

• *The problem of female life expectancy in South Asia.* Female life expectancy is longer than male life expectancy in all countries of the world except in three South Asian countries: Bangladesh, India, and Nepal. The seriousness of this problem cannot be overemphasized. In the other Asian countries, women live two to seven years longer than men (table 7.1). Thus the life expectancy of women in South Asia may be depressed by four years, or nearly 10 percent of their lives. At the level of aggregation used in this study, it appears that most of the deficit is related to problems in the childbearing years, but other studies have found that the deficit starts in infancy and persists through middle age. Ratios of population by sex, for example, tend to favor men across most age groups in India. Assuming that this problem arises from allocations of resources in the home away from women,[1] do government allocations offset the misallocation in any way? We have found little or no evidence that there is any offset, as attested to by the rudimentary development of maternal and child health services in South Asia.

Governments in all three South Asian countries have population policies that commit them to reducing population growth; however, the effectiveness of family planning efforts must be hindered if there is a lack of complementary health services for women in their childbearing years. Although the anomaly of shorter life expectancy for women is exceptional by both world and Asian standards, it was shared by Sri Lanka in the 1940s and was reversed quickly in that country when health conditions began to improve in the early 1950s; in fact, it appears to have been a major component of the improvement.

Differences in performance, 1965-86. Although all countries in the Asian sample have seen improvements in life expectancy in the last 20 years, two of the countries with the worst indicators in 1965, Bangladesh and Nepal, fell further behind by 1986 because of slower-than-average improvements. Life expectancy in the Philippines and Thailand also improved at a slower rate than for the sample as a whole. Although the slowness of the improvement in the high-mortality countries is a major concern, the slowing of changes in middle-income countries, such as the Philippines and Thailand, cannot be blamed on low incomes, but suggest possible problems in health policy. If those two countries had kept up with average improvements in life expectancy for the sample over the period, female life expectancy today would stand at 68 years in the Philippines and 70 years in Thailand, a considerable improvement over the figures in table 7.1 (65 and 66 years, respectively).

As a result of the uneven performance among the Asian countries, countries with the highest mortality rates were in a worse relative position in 1986 than in 1965, and some countries, such as the Philippines, fell behind countries that had similar health indicators in 1965. For example, Bangladesh's infant mortality rate in 1965 was approximately 2.8 times higher than Malaysia's. By 1986 Bangladesh's rate was 4.5 times Malaysia's. The Philippines fell behind China and Thailand over the period, and Myanmar is rapidly catching up with it.

Health, demography, and health financing

A review of the evidence on mortality and demographic changes in the Asian countries provides some general guidelines for thinking about health policy. For countries with shorter life expectancies (the first group in table 7.1), improvements in the future will be tied closely to success in reducing both infant mortality and the female mortality differential. Targeting the birth process (including family planning) will tend to improve outcomes for both women and children.

Statistics on causes of death point to the continuing importance of infectious and parasitic diseases in developing countries for all age groups. Targeting infectious and parasitic diseases will reinforce the effect of targeting the birth process for children in the younger age groups, but it will also reduce death rates in all other age groups. The evidence suggests that if countries in this sample can reduce deaths due to infectious diseases and other or unknown causes (even in countries with low mortality rates), death rates in all age groups can fall to levels close to those achieved in industrial countries even if mortality due to chronic disease problems does *not* fall significantly. Reducing the incidence of infectious and parasitic diseases will have payoffs across the age spectrum and will not be captured by a single group, but greater public resources devoted to chronic disease problems would tend to be captured by older groups (over age 45).

The recent literature emphasizing adult health problems has argued that chronic disease problems will begin to dominate the mortality profiles of countries that have succeeded in increasing their life expectancy over the last two decades. Although it is true that, in percentage terms, the group over age 65 will be the fastest growing in many Asian countries, fast growth in a relatively small group still leaves it a relatively small group. Only in China and Korea will less than 75 percent of the population be under 45 years of age in 2005, and in both countries the group over age 65 will still be less than 10 percent of the population. Moreover, members of the oldest group are much more likely to die of infectious and parasitic diseases than are their counterparts in industrial countries. The 0-4 age group will actually be shrinking in about half the sample, but it is so large in absolute terms that small percentage reductions will leave it quite large. Only in Korea will the 0-14 age group make up less than 25 percent of the population in 2005. Almost all of the health problems in that group are concentrated in the first year or two of life. In fact, the age structure of the population in 2005 brings the promise of healthier populations as today's large bulge of youngsters moves into the middle-aged groups and as women have fewer children.

The immediate challenge posed by demographic changes in Asian countries is quite different from that emphasized in the adult health and epidemiological transition literatures. It is the huge increase in the number of women of childbearing age in most countries, caused by persistently high population growth rates over the last several decades. Except in the very low-mortality and low-fertility countries, this group will increase as a share of the population to nearly a quarter by 2005. These women will have fewer children, they will be more urbanized, they will have more education, and they will use more health services than were available to their mothers. They are the main group to benefit from family planning. About half the women in this cohort are now school-age children, and one of the most effective health interventions they or their future children will ever receive is being provided through their schools. The investments being made in these young women today and the services they use during their childbearing years will strongly affect the health of the 25 to 40 percent of the population under age 15 in 2005. In the countries of South Asia, inadequate attention to the health and education of this group today is a portent of poor performance in the health sector over the next several decades.

Health systems and patterns of expenditure

The mean for health expenditure as a percentage of GNP in the Asian sample is 3.1 percent, somewhat less than half of the 7 to 8 percent of GNP spent on health in industrial countries. In absolute dollar amounts, this share of GNP translates into less than 3 percent of the health spending in the industrial countries.

Korea, whose total spending on health stands at about 5 percent of GNP, spends about 1 percent more of its GNP on health care than does its nearest rival, India (figure 7.1). Six countries—China, India, Malaysia, Myanmar, Papua New Guinea, and Thailand—spend more than 3 percent of their GNP on health. This group is a disparate collection of low-income and middle-income countries, with no particular pattern reflected in the size or composition of their expenditures. The group that spends the least on health—less than 2 percent of GNP—includes the countries with the worst health indicators—Bangladesh and Nepal.

Figure 7.1 Health expenditure by source as a percentage of GNP, in selected Asian countries, most recent year

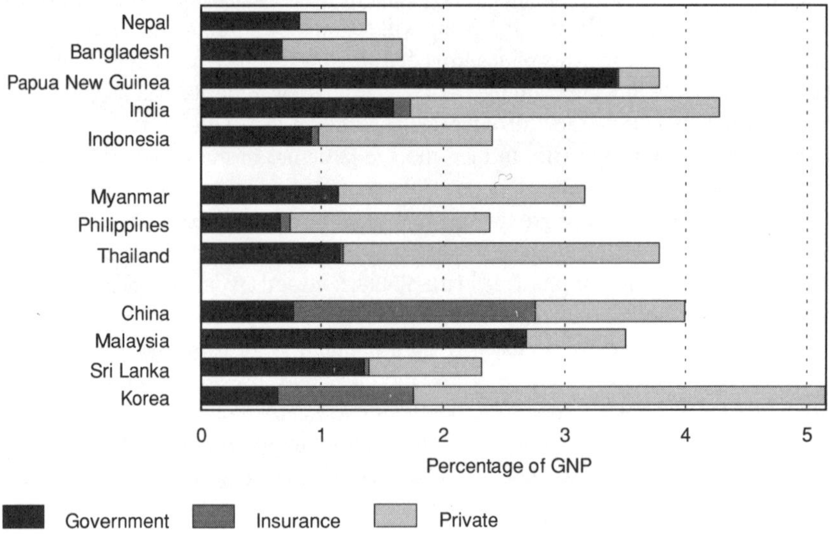

Source: Appendix table A.9.

Public spending accounts for more than half of total spending in Malaysia, Nepal, Papua New Guinea, and Sri Lanka (figure 7.1). Private out-of-pocket expenditure plays an important role in all countries, but in Bangladesh, India, Indonesia, Korea, Myanmar, the Philippines, and Thailand private spending accounts for more than half the total. Insurance financing, or some form of third-party payment system, is poorly developed except in China and Korea, where insurance appears to displace a substantial amount of direct government spending. Conversely, countries with a high proportion of government spending, including Malaysia and Papua New Guinea, tend not to have developed third-party payment systems.

In the more *revenue-constrained* countries, such as Bangladesh, Nepal, Indonesia, and the Philippines, which would benefit from higher spending on health by government and the diversion of public resources out of curative services, user fees may provide an attractive alternative to full government financing of curative services in the state health system. Because of the high incidence of poverty, any such fee strategy would require careful targeting of the remaining government subsidies to the neediest. Greater dependence on the private sector and on private-public partnerships to deliver care holds promise for improving the operational efficiency of the health systems to free up resources in existing budgets. That is particularly true in Bangladesh, which is training large numbers of physicians that the public sector cannot absorb. Insurance or risk-sharing options are not important for either Bangladesh or Nepal, although insurance for formal sector (government) employees would start the development of the necessary institutional structures and create a mechanism through which those who are best off would pay for their own health care.

Indonesia and the Philippines are considered revenue-constrained because of their low public spending on health, which is not completely compensated for by the private sector. The private sector is well developed in both countries, and the governments invest heavily in hospitals despite relatively low public sector spending. Higher spending on public health activities, coupled with efforts to reduce the burden of curative services on the public budget—greater cost recovery in clinics and hospitals, less duplication of private sector activities, and greater attention to insurance—would increase economic efficiency in the sector and allow these two governments to retarget their health expenditures to a more appropriate combination of activities. Although both countries could absorb considerably more government spending on health, they also must use existing expenditures more effectively. They enjoy a much higher level of development than Bangladesh and Nepal, so they are less constrained by exogenous forces (low incomes, low educational achievement) in formulating health policy.

Countries with *relatively high private and public spending*, including India, Myanmar, and Thailand, are less constrained by resources and may have little interest in adjusting their policies. However, the development of insurance in those countries is probably desirable from the client's viewpoint, given their current high private expenditures. Greater attention to insurance is also sensible from the standpoint of public welfare: disease patterns are likely to change rapidly in the future in these countries, leading to greater demands for chronic care and the expensive hospital-based technologies that it requires. In each country, the government remains heavily involved in the provision of hospital services, which insurance is best suited to finance.

India's relatively high spending on health as a percentage of GNP, much of which is out-of-pocket spending by individuals and decentralized spending by state governments, raises some policy questions unique to its situation. Is the relatively small share of spending controlled by the central government devoted to urgent priorities that are not getting adequate attention at either the state or the household level? Two of the most important health issues are the relatively poor health outcomes for women up to age 45 and persistently high infant mortality in some areas of the country. Are central government funds channeled into these areas? Are public health activities the first priority for these funds? The evidence suggests that the allocation of central government funds does not target these persistent problems. The largest single component of the central health budget is medical education: maternal and child health services receive only 20 percent of the amount the central government spends to train physicians. India's extraordinary level of public funding for hospitals makes it an outlier for its level of income and health status; this priority seems unwarranted. India's relatively high spending creates many opportunities in the health sector; better allocation of existing resources might allow it to match China's performance in the sector.

Three countries, Malaysia, Papua New Guinea, and, to a lesser degree, Sri Lanka, *have high total expenditure on health that comes largely from the public sector*. Such expenditure patterns may be the result of carefully considered decisions and government priorities in those countries; thus there may be little desire or felt need to change the sources of revenue. But there is little question, given the experience of the other countries in the sample, that some part of this high public spending does little more than substitute for private expenditure that would be made anyway, either out of pocket or through insurance. Because these countries have exceptionally high spending, there is wide scope (economically, if not politically) for adjustments in how the sector is financed and how the government targets its own spending. All three countries are, in fact, exploring some of the possibilities.

Finally, China and Korea have *high total expenditure, low direct government expenditure, and relatively heavy dependence on insurance financing*. They are rapidly moving into the policy problems faced by industrial countries—cost containment, rationing of medical care, optimal reimbursement methods, and how to plan better for health sector investments under decentralized third-party payment systems. In both countries the public role is complex because the government is largely in the background, exercising relatively little direct control over the delivery of services and confining itself to a policymaking and financial role. Many important public decisions in both countries are not so much direct spending decisions as they are indirect allocation decisions (such as reimbursement policies) that affect the sector through the behavioral reactions of providers and hospital administrators. These decisions require good information and highly trained managers. In addition, it is important that public health aspects of government spending not lose priority. Recent health policy studies by the World Bank in China and Korea have emphasized the persistent public health issues underlying the problems of chronic disease that are beginning to surface in both countries. The financing mechanisms used in China and Korea may prove to perform poorly in making cost-effective allocations to manage these problems, creating a new challenge to policy that other countries in the region will also face eventually.

Equity issues: Patterns in the targeting of government expenditure

Government spending accounts for less than half of health sector spending in all but five countries (figure 7.1). But the government is the most important spending authority in the sector, and the allocation of public health resources can have a significant effect on health outcomes, especially in poorer countries, where most of the health problems *are* public health problems. The effects of government health spending on equity thus fall into two broad areas.

First, is the government targeting its spending to areas of the country with high mortality? If vectors transmitting disease are controlled (important for malaria, schistosomiasis, and many other parasitic diseases), and the communication of waterborne diseases is managed through safe water and sanitation, there is little question that health will improve largely independent of changes in individual behavior.[2] Moreover, such interventions as control of communicable diseases, provision of adequate drinking water and sewerage facilities, and regulation of air and water pollution can benefit the poor relatively more than the rich, if only because the poor are less able to compensate for inadequate public investments in these areas. Almost as important is the fact that investments in public goods can usually be targeted geographically—for example, to impoverished areas and disadvantaged population groups. Curative budgets can be targeted in the same way. Targeting public expenditure by geographical differences in infant mortality may in fact be an excellent way to target the poor.

Second, there is little expectation that private sector or insurance expenditures will benefit the poor, so in terms of redistribution, the government is virtually the only player in the health sector. If the government fails to target its spending to the poor, no other source of funds is likely to compensate for that failure to any important degree.

This report considers methods governments could use to improve the targeting of health spending, but it also examines in some detail how government expenditure patterns for a subset of the sample are related to regional differences in per capita income and infant mortality. The underlying presumption in this exercise is that governments interested in targeting some portion of health spending to the poor and reducing infant mortality would target areas that have lower per capita incomes and higher infant mortality.

The findings are not encouraging. In India, for example, where state (rather than central) government resources make up the bulk of total public health resources (86 percent), it is probably to be expected that state-level health spending is higher in states that are richer and in those that have lower infant mortality rates. That turns out to be the case. However, even though the central government targets a small share of its expenditure to the poorer parts of the country, overall central government spending appears not to be targeted effectively to the poorest areas and those with the worst health indicators. India's urban residents, for example, capture a share of the total public health expenditure nearly 2.5 times larger than their share in the population. Central government allocations are negatively related to state infant mortality rates, contrary to what might be expected on either health or redistributive grounds. Furthermore, despite India's strong commitment to family planning and its high female mortality rate, maternal and child health programs are in only a rudimentary stage of development. For the most part, public spending is funneled through curative institutions.

Bangladesh has the unusual record of having retargeted spending toward rural areas in the last decade, but because overall spending is so low, the result has been a dilution of the quality of government health services and difficulty in channelling available subsidies to lower-income groups. It is widely believed that usage rates at public rural clinics have dropped as people have sought non-government services because of the low quality and poor functioning of the public facilities. A fundamental flaw in the retargeting effort appears to lie in the failure to reorient spending away from curative toward preventive health services and to provide significant net additions to total spending.

In Indonesia and Papua New Guinea central government spending also benefits better-off groups. In Papua New Guinea, for example, the National Capital District absorbs a disproportionately large share of the sector's total resources even though it has the lowest rate of infant mortality. The reason, of course, is the high spending on the large national hospital located there, which draws most of its clients from only a small geographic area. Outside the District, allocations of health spending through government facilities also favor better-off areas, but the bias is offset almost completely by the religious missions through which some government funds are spent. This experience points to a potential role for charitable organizations as a conduit of public resources to the rural poor.

Finally, in Malaysia, alone among the other countries for which the geographical distribution of expenditure could be determined, the lowest-income groups appear to capture a fair share of total public spending on health, and spending across localities shows a flat rather than a positive link to incomes. The Malaysian experience suggests that it is possible to avoid biases against the poor in the allocation of public health resources. Even so, if Malaysia is the best performer in the region and its spending is merely flat across income and mortality groups, there is much room for improvement.

One would in fact expect to see a negative relation between government health spending and income and a positive relation between government health spending and infant mortality rates. It is difficult to characterize current public policies as redistributive and oriented to health problems when they redistribute to areas that are better off financially and target healthier populations.

Although this effort to identify distributive consequences of health spending is rudimentary and depends on old data in some cases, the findings suggest that there is wide scope for better targeting both of people and of diseases in this sample of countries. The targeting need not take the form of subsidies for curative care, although those may be appropriate in some countries. China, Korea, and Malaysia have shown that intensive provision of public health interventions can have tremendous effects on such measures of health as infant mortality. These effects can be accomplished in large part with inexpensive local inputs, and they benefit the poor at least as much as the rich.

Research priorities

Research priorities resulting from this study are driven by what we do not know or could not uncover. A top priority must be to subject population programs to the same type of analysis. It was attempted as part of this study, but putting together financial statistics for population programs that are comparable across countries appears to be virtually impossible without spending considerable time poring over budget documents and reports from each country. It is a time-consuming but important task to carry out.

A second major hole in the data is a lack of cost information on some basic features of health systems: wages, prices of such inputs as drugs and medical supplies, capital costs, and the costs of training personnel. The conventional wisdom on the organization of health services in developing countries is based almost entirely on a view of what is technically appropriate to certain health conditions. We know almost nothing about what is economically appropriate based on local costs of inputs and resources. Basic information on costs and prices should be collected regularly to assist in planning both at the country level and by donors.

A third problem is a nearly incapacitating lack of knowledge about how government budgets are distributed between public health activities and curative health activities. The public-private distinction is the most important functional classification that can be made for government budgets from both an economic and a public health perspective, thus it is extraordinary that it is almost never made in public budgets.

We need much better knowledge of the public health problems that people face. These problems vary by location—urban or rural—and by environmental characteristics. Countries almost need a "health map" to lay out priorities for public spending, but such information is almost entirely lacking. Once the public health problems are known, we need cost-benefit analysis (at best) or cost-effectiveness analysis (at least) to determine quantitatively which methods would be most appropriate economically and how to establish priorities among competing needs. This area requires funding for focused research projects and the development of skills necessary to carry out the work on a regular basis as part of a ministry of health's normal operations. It should also become an integral part of donor-financed health projects.

A fourth research priority is for governments to better understand who captures subsidies provided through the health sector. In this study, a very rough and aggregative approach is attempted in the equity chapter, but that can be only a start on what needs to be done. A rigorous approach to equity issues requires household and community surveys. We must also understand much better the connection between gender and health spending in order to understand better how to offset household allocation decisions that create public health problems, such as the female health deficit in South Asia.

Fifth, the major financing issues from a demand side are related to user fees and, for about half the countries in this sample, how to expand insurance coverage either through the public or the private sector. There is a concern that fee and insurance policies disregard equity problems and public health activities; in fact, insurance and fees in the health sector are integral parts of the solution to all of these problems. Any policy that affects the behavior of clients and providers—fees and insurance certainly do, but so do any service delivery decisions that depend on client behavior for success—must be planned and carried out with some knowledge of their behavior. Further work in fees and insurance requires careful design of household and provider surveys to guide policy changes. Beyond that, technical expertise in the planning and carrying out of structural and administrative changes required for fees and insurance, and expertise in designing such systems so that they do not unduly distort incentives, are also necessary. In most of Asia, and within the World Bank, this is virgin territory. The Bank should build capacity now to help developing countries meet the coming challenges in the financing of curative health care. In fact, that is the main challenge in the transition from high- to low-mortality environments—how to finance curative care in a low-income setting in an equitable and efficient manner.

Finally, Bank projects should be designed to help answer some of the outstanding empirical questions—questions about appropriate interactions of the public and private sectors, the effectiveness of means-testing programs and methods to reach the poor, alternative approaches to solving public health problems—that require both experimentation and analysis. There is a need to try innovative programs of user fees; fee retention at facilities; conversion of public to private facilities; innovative cooperative efforts between the public and private sectors; rural insurance schemes; and even "negative user fees" (subsidies or gifts) to attract some groups, such as pregnant women in South Asia, into the health system. These activities require a combination of informed planning, operations work, and rigorous evaluation. Cost analysis will play a major role in all such efforts, but the focus must be on alternative approaches that adjust to local conditions (including prices and incomes), rather than on a single "medically correct" approach.

Overall conclusions

There are dangers in drawing specific conclusions from this broad compendium of material. Generalizations necessarily disregard the widely divergent institutional contexts that help to shape policy in each country, and the numbers on which the analysis is based are imprecise. Yet some basic themes have surfaced repeatedly even in this short summary.

While Asia as a whole has performed well in health and fertility relative to other regions in the world, the performance within the region has been almost divergent enough to render the regional average meaningless. The countries in the region that have performed well in health and fertility differ from their neighbors today partly because of policy decisions and allocations they have made in the health sector in the past. It follows that the handful of countries that have lagged behind the group have done so because of decisions they have made, particularly about spending *levels* in the health sector. Moreover, the countries that have not performed well have made *allocation* decisions that may have compounded the problem of low spending. These countries, including Bangladesh, Nepal, Indonesia, and the Philippines, would probably benefit from both greater spending in the health sector and a review of spending priorities.

A second important finding is that the financial base that most countries in the sample have tapped to finance government health services is narrow. Although there are three possible sources of revenue (taxes, insurance, and private spending), most government systems depend almost completely on tax revenues. There are many opportunities to broaden the health sector's financial base through user fees and insurance, as China and Korea have done. Because most countries in the sample already have relatively large private sectors, pluralistic systems exist that the government can tap into, probably with only minor changes in policy. Malaysia and Papua New Guinea, in contrast, have chosen to spend so heavily out of tax revenues for health care that they have probably supplanted private spending and hindered the development of insurance. However, both countries have had success with their approach and therefore provide an example for other countries that prefer that route.

A third finding flows from the effort to compare government spending with common ideas of fairness about what governments should do with their money. One of the hypotheses investigated here is that governments interested in equity would allocate more resources to poorer areas. They do not—at least that is the message from the small number of countries for which data could be assembled. The best performer, Malaysia, achieves flat spending across the range of incomes that characterize its political subdivisions. The second idea investigated was that governments would spend more money in political subdivisions with higher infant mortality rates. They do not—at least for the countries investigated in this project. Better targeting is certainly feasible and desirable on both counts.

By far the most striking finding is the reaffirmation in the available data of the continuing importance of the same infectious and parasitic diseases that have been killing people in Asia for centuries. This situation requires governments to orient themselves toward improving public health programs—not adult health programs or old-age programs, but programs that give children a healthy start in life and ensure that their lives will be lived in environments relatively free from life-threatening or debilitating diseases that can be prevented. All age and income groups will benefit from greater control over communicable diseases. The emphasis on public health increases as countries are poorer, spend less on health, and have worse health outcomes. In this area there is a good fit between an economic approach to the sector and the work of public health professionals. There is a poor fit between what should be done and what many governments actually do. A related and somewhat surprising finding is the persistence of high mortality for women in South Asia—even as we approach the 21st century, and after decades of mortality decline—and the poorly developed public policies to solve the problem.

The allocation of spending between public health and curative health poses an issue of political economy. Competition for public resources in the health sector tends to be dominated by those who can derive the most direct benefit from them—hospital administrators, physicians, and nurses. As these groups succeed in competing for public resources to make their activities more effective, public spending will be diverted toward curative care interventions.

In contrast, because everyone benefits more or less equally from effective public health programs, any single person's benefit is so small relative to a physician's salary or a hospital administrator's budget that little direct support for public health benefits is generated by the self-interest of beneficiaries. Moreover, when a person becomes ill with malaria, he or she has a strong interest in curative care; when not ill with malaria, the person has no equally intense interest in public policies to prevent it. Accordingly, advocacy for public health spending tends to be voluntary, poorly organized, and intermittent. Donors must take care not to fall into the same patterns of spending that are created by internal pressures on developing country governments. Rather, donors should take a strong advocacy position for public health activities. The litmus test of success for any policy-based lending in the health sector should thus be improved public health activities and the creation of institutional advocates for public health (such as schools of public health, a large component of public health training for government physicians, and relatively large public health divisions in the government with statistical and policymaking functions).

Notes

1. And implicitly, away from children around birth.
2. Although changes in behavior would complement these changes in environment.

Appendix

Table A.1 Basic economic indicators and regions used in calculations for chapter 2, mid-1980s

Region/country	*Population*	*GNP per capita*	*GNP*	*GDP*	*Consumption (percent)*	*Government consumption (percent)*
2 Ethiopia	43.5	120	5220	4960	80	17
1 Bhutan	1.3	150	195	210	..	..
2 Burkina Faso	8.1	150	1215	930	91	15
1 Nepal	17	150	2550	2200	84	8
1 Bangladesh	103.2	160	16512	15460	90	8
2 Malawi	7.4	160	1184	1100	75	18
2 Zaire	31.7	160	5072	6020	81	7
2 Mali	7.6	180	1368	1650	83	13
1 Myanmar	38	200	7600	8180	74	14
2 Mozambique	14.2	210	2982	4300	86	15
2 Madagascar	10.6	230	2438	2670	76	13
2 Uganda	15.2	230	3496	3310	89	..
2 Burundi	4.8	240	1152	1090	79	12
2 Tanzania	23	250	5750	4020	89	8
2 Togo	3.1	250	775	980	71	15
2 Niger	6.6	260	1716	2080	82	11
2 Benin	4.2	270	1134	1320	90	9
2 Somalia	5.5	280	1540	2320	93	12
2 Central African Rep.	2.7	290	783	900	88	9
1 India	781.4	290	226606	203790	67	12
2 Rwanda	6.2	290	1798	1850	71	20
1 China	1054	300	316200	271880	50	14
2 Kenya	21.2	300	6360	5960	55	19
2 Zambia	6.9	300	2070	1660	62	25
2 Sierra Leone	3.8	310	1178	1180	92	..
2 Sudan	22.6	320	7232	7470	83	14
4 Haiti	6.1	330	2013	2150	83	12
3 Pakistan	99.2	350	34720	30080	81	12
2 Lesotho	1.6	370	592	230	143	35
2 Ghana	13.2	390	5148	5720	82	10
1 Sri Lanka	16.1	400	6440	5880	78	9
2 Mauritania	1.8	420	756	750	71	14
2 Senegal	6.8	420	2856	3740	77	17
3 Afghanistan	19.2	..	..	..	..	..
2 Chad	5.1	..	..	..	..	..
2 Guinea	6.3	..	..	1980	73	14
1 Kampuchea	7.9	..	..	..	..	..
1 Lao PDR	3.7	..	..	..	..	..
1 Viet Nam	63.3	..	..	..	..	..
2 Liberia	2.3	460	1058	990	65	17

Medical care consumption	Central government health, % of budget	Government exp. as % of GNP	Total health spending per capita	Central government health spending per capita	Approximate private health spending per capita
..	..	..	3.32	..	..
..	..	..	..	..	..
..	6.2	13.2	..	1.23	..
..	5	19.7	..	1.48	..
..	5.3	10.9	..	0.92	..
3	6.9	31.5	4.15	3.48	0.67
3	..	..	5.01	..	..
1	1.7	34	2.08	1.04	1.04
..	7.7	16.2	..	2.49	..
..	..	..	..	..	..
1	..	..		2.24	..
..	2.4	9.4	..	0.52	..
..	..	..	..	..	..
1	4.9	23.9	1.7	2.93	..
.	3.6	42.3	..	3.81	..
..	..	..	..	..	..
5	..	..	15.56	..	..
..	..	..	..	..	..
..	..	..	..	..	..
3	2.1	16.4	6.18	1	5.18
4	..	..	10.86	..	..
..	..	..	..	..	..
..	6.4	27.8	..	5.34	..
5	7.2	38.2	10.47	8.25	2.21
2	5.8	13.6	..	2.45	..
6	..	..	19.24	..	..
..	..	..	..	..	..
3	1	23.1	8.46	0.81	7.65
..	6.9	24.2	..	6.18	..
3	8.3	14	11.96	4.53	7.43
3	4	30.5	9.53	4.88	4.65
..	..	..	..	..	..
2	..	..	10.34	..	..
..	..	..	..	..	..
..	..	..	..	..	..
..	..	..	..	..	..
..	..	..	..	..	..
..	..	..	..	..	..
..	..	..	..	..	..
..	5.7	27.1	..	7.11	..

Table A.1 Basic economic indicators and regions used in calculations for chapter 2, mid-1980s (cont.)

Region/country	*Population*	*GNP per capita*	*GNP*	*GDP*	*Consumption (percent)*	*Government consumption (percent)*
3 Yemen PDR	2.2	470	1034	930	..	..
1 Indonesia	166.4	490	81536	75230	64	12
3 Yemen Arab Rep.	8.2	550	4510	4760	93	22
1 Philippines	57.3	560	32088	30540	73	8
3 Morocco	22.5	590	13275	14760	70	17
4 Bolivia	6.6	600	3960	4180	85	10
2 Zimbabwe	8.7	620	5394	4940	62	19
2 Nigeria	103.1	640	65984	49110	78	12
4 Dominican Rep.	6.6	710	4686	5280	80	8
1 Papua New Guinea	3.4	720	2448	2530	63	22
2 Côte d'Ivoire	10.7	730	7811	7320	62	15
4 Honduras	4.5	740	3330	2960	70	17
3 Egypt	49.7	760	37772	40850	72	19
4 Nicaragua	3.4	790	2686	2900	57	45
1 Thailand	52.6	810	42606	41780	62	13
4 El Salvador	4.9	820	4018	3980	79	14
2 Botswana	1.1	840	924	1150	47	28
4 Jamaica	2.4	840	2016	2430	65	15
2 Cameroon	10.5	910	9555	11280	62	9
4 Guatemala	8.2	930	7626	7470	84	7
2 Congo	2	990	1980	2000	50	20
4 Paraguay	3.8	1000	3800	3590	87	7
4 Peru	19.8	1090	21582	25370	71	11
3 Turkey	51.5	1110	57165	52620	69	9
3 Tunisia	7.3	1140	8322	7790	66	17
4 Ecuador	9.6	1160	11136	11510	68	12
2 Mauritius	1	1200	1200	1160	64	11
4 Colombia	29	1230	35670	29660	68	12
4 Chile	12.2	1320	16104	16820	69	13
4 Costa Rica	2.6	1480	3848	4260	59	17
3 Jordan	3.6	1540	5544	4000	81	27
3 Syria	10.8	1570	16956	17400	62	25
3 Lebanon	2.8	..	..	..	..	..
4 Brazil	138.4	1810	250504	206750	76	..
1 Malaysia	16.1	1830	29463	27580	51	17
2 South Africa	32.3	1850	59755	56370	51	19
4 Mexico	80.2	1860	149172	127140	64	10
4 Uruguay	3	1900	5700	5320	73	14
3 Hungary	10.6	2020	21412	23660	65	10
3 Poland	38.5	2070	79695	73770	70	..

Medical care consumption	*Central government health, % of budget*	*Government exp. as % of GNP*	*Total health spending per capita*	*Central government health spending per capita*	*Approximate private health spending per capita*
..	..	..	..	..	..
2	1.9	26.9	6.87	2.5	4.37
..	4.7	25.5	..	6.59	..
4	6	10.8	17.27	3.63	13.64
3	2.8	35.3	17.12	5.83	11.29
5	1.4	32	30.08	2.69	27.4
..	6.2	35.2	..	13.53	..
3	..	..	12.86	..	..
8	9	15.3	56.32	9.78	46.54
..	9.6	34.8	..	24.05	..
1	4	31.2	5.27	9.11	..
8	..	..	45.78	..	..
14	2.4	40.6	104.71	7.41	97.31
..	..	56.4	..	..	..
6	5.7	21.7	35.74	10.02	25.72
8	7.5	12.9	60.43	7.93	52.5
4	5	49.4	31.36	20.75	10.62
3	..	..	24.3	..	..
7	5.1	22.4	53.39	10.4	43
13	..	..	107.77	..	..
22	..	..	154	..	..
2	3.1	7.9	17.76	2.45	15.31
4	..	14.1	42.03	..	..
4	2.2	21.8	31.88	5.32	26.55
3	6.5	36.9	26.57	27.34	..
5	7.3	15.7	47.96	13.29	34.66
13	7.7	24.9	113.1	23.01	90.09
7	..	..	57.27	..	..
5	6	33.6	56.53	26.61	29.92
7	19.3	29.3	87.17	83.69	3.47
5	3.8	46	60	26.92	33.08
..	..	..	..	..	..
..	..	..	..	..	..
6	6.4	26.4	..	30.58	..
5	..	36.6	58.24	..	..
..	..	26.8	..	..	..
5	1.4	27.3	58.66	7.11	51.55
6	4.8	24.7	92.57	22.53	70.04
5	3.6	62.6	83.7	45.52	38.18
6	..	42.2	..	..	..

Table A.1 Basic economic indicators and regions used in calculations for chapter 2, mid-1980s (cont.)

Region/country	*Population*	*GNP per capita*	*GNP*	*GDP*	*Consumption (percent)*	*Government consumption (percent)*
3 Portugal	10.2	2250	22950	27480	66	14
3 Yugoslavia	23.3	2300	53590	61640	46	14
4 Panama	2.2	2330	5126	5120	57	22
4 Argentina	31	2350	72850	69820	77	12
1 Korea, Rep.	41.5	2370	98355	98150	55	10
3 Algeria	22.4	2590	58016	60760	69	..
4 Venezuela	17.8	2920	51976	49980	66	13
2 Gabon	1	3080	3080	3190	55	26
5 Greece	10	3680	36800	35210	66	19
3 Oman	1.3	4950	6435	7320	..	..
4 Trinidad and Tobago	1.2	5360	6432	4830	62	19
3 Israel	4.3	6210	26703	29460	58	31
1 Hong Kong	5.4	6910	37314	32250	65	8
1 Singapore	2.6	7410	19266	18350	48	12
3 Iran	45.6	..	..	..	..	..
3 Iraq	16.5	..	..	..	..	..
3 Romania	22.9	..	..	..	..	..
3 Saudi Arabia	12	6950	83400	78480	43	40
3 Kuwait	1.8	13890	25002	22310	..	..
3 United Arab Emirates	1.4	14680	20552	25280	..	..
3 Libya	3.9	..	..	..	..	..
5 Spain	38.7	4860	188082	229100	63	14
5 Ireland	3.6	5070	18252	21910	58	19
5 New Zealand	3.3	7460	24618	26630	60	16
5 Italy	57.2	8550	489060	599920	61	16
5 United Kingdom	56.7	8870	502929	468290	62	21
5 Belgium	9.9	9230	91377	112180	64	17
5 Austria	7.6	9990	75924	93830	56	19
5 Netherlands	14.6	10020	146292	175330	59	16
5 France	55.4	10720	593888	724200	61	19
5 Australia	16	11920	190720	184940	61	19
5 Germany, Fed. Rep.	60.9	12080	735672	891990	56	20
5 Finland	4.9	12160	59584	62370	55	21
5 Denmark	5.1	12600	64260	68820	55	24
5 Japan	121.5	12840	1560060	1955650	58	10
5 Sweden	8.4	13160	110544	114470	52	27
5 Canada	25.6	14120	361472	323790	58	20
5 Norway	4.2	15400	64680	69780	54	20
5 United States	241.6	17480	4223168	4185490	66	19
5 Switzerland	6.5	17680	114920	135050	60	13

.. Not available.
Source: See table A.5.

Medical care consumption	Central government health, % of budget	Government exp. as % of GNP	Total health spending per capita	Central government health spending per capita	Approximate private health spending per capita
6	..	..	129.32	..	..
6	..	6.6	95.24	..	..
8	15.8	32.5	147.08	119.65	27.44
4	1.3	25.8	80.18	7.88	72.3
4	1.5	17.8	61.49	6.33	55.16
..	..	..	..	..	..
8	8.1	26.6	177.46	62.91	114.54
..	..	41	..	..	..
6	..	50.9	179.57	..	..
..	5	63.2	..	156.42	..
..	..	..	..	..	..
6	3.4	72.1	365.85	152.23	213.62
6	..	..	261.58	..	..
7	6.5	26.5	296.42	127.64	168.79
..	..	..	..	..	..
..	..	..	..	..	..
..	0.8	..	..	..	..
..	..	..	..	..	..
..	7.1	41.5	..	409.27	..
..	6.2	17.5	..	159.28	..
..	..	..	..	..	..
7	13.1	29.1	319.08	185.27	133.81
10	13.2	54.7	468.63	366.07	102.56
9	12.5	42.8	551.97	399.11	152.86
10	9.9	50.2	807.58	424.92	382.67
8	12.6	40.6	548.4	453.75	94.65
10	1.7	56.7	917.84	88.97	828.87
10	12	40.5	925.95	485.51	440.44
11	10.8	56.6	990.73	612.5	378.23
13	..	44.1	1359.51	..	..
10	9.5	27.9	924.7	315.94	608.76
13	17.9	29.9	1447.1	646.53	800.57
9	10.6	31.1	870.63	400.87	469.77
8	1	39.5	852.83	49.77	803.06
10	..	17.4	1094.52	..	..
11	1.1	44.1	1184.22	63.84	1120.38
5	6.1	25.4	493.27	218.78	274.5
10	10.5	40.6	1229.46	656.5	572.96
14	11.6	24.6	2061.56	498.81	1562.75
15	13.1	18.6	2275.07	430.79	1844.28

Table A.2 Health indicators used in calculations for chapter 2, mid-1980s

Country	Female life expectancy 1965	Female life expectancy 1986	% change in female life exp. 1965–86	Male life expectancy 1965	Male life expectancy 1986	% change in male life exp. 1965–86
Ethiopia	43	48	11.63	42	45	7.14
Bhutan	32	45	40.63	30	46	53.33
Burkina Faso	40	49	22.5	37	45	21.62
Nepal	40	47	17.5	41	48	17.07
Bangladesh	44	50	13.64	45	51	13.33
Malawi	40	47	17.5	39	44	12.82
Zaire	45	54	20	42	50	19.05
Mali	39	48	23.08	37	45	21.62
Myanmar	49	61	24.49	46	58	26.09
Mozambique	39	49	25.64	36	46	27.78
Madagascar	45	55	22.22	42	52	23.81
Uganda	47	49	4.26	44	46	4.55
Burundi	45	50	11.11	42	47	11.9
Tanzania	45	55	22.22	41	51	24.39
Togo	44	54	22.73	40	51	27.5
Niger	39	46	17.95	35	43	22.86
Benin	43	52	20.93	41	48	17.07
Somalia	40	48	20	37	45	21.62
Central African Rep.	41	51	24.39	40	48	20
India	44	56	27.27	46	57	23.91
Rwanda	51	50	-1.96	47	47	0
China	56	70	25	50	68	36
Kenya	50	59	18	46	56	21.74
Zambia	46	54	17.39	43	51	18.6
Sierra Leone	34	42	23.53	31	40	29.03
Sudan	41	51	24.39	39	47	20.51
Haiti	47	56	19.15	44	53	20.45
Pakistan	44	51	15.91	46	52	13.04
Lesotho	50	57	14	47	53	12.77
Ghana	49	56	14.29	46	52	13.04
Sri Lanka	65	72	10.77	63	68	7.94
Mauritania	39	49	25.64	36	45	25
Senegal	42	49	16.67	40	46	15
Afghanistan	35	..	..	35	..	..
Chad	38	46	21.05	35	44	25.71
Guinea	36	43	19.44	34	41	20.59
Kampuchea	46	..	..	43	..	..
Lao PDR	..	51	..	..	48	..
Viet Nam	..	68	..	..	63	..
Liberia	46	56	21.74	43	52	20.93
Yemen PDR	39	51	30.77	38	49	28.95

Female minus male life expectancy 1986	Female change minus male change in life expectancy	Infant mortality rate 1965	Infant mortality rate 1986	% change in IMR 1965–86
3	4.49	165	155	-6.06
-1	-12.71	184	139	-24.5
4	0.88	193	140	-27.5
-1	0.43	184	130	-29.4
-1	0.3	153	121	-20.9
3	4.68	200	153	-23.5
4	0.95	141	100	-29.1
3	1.46	207	144	-30.4
3	-1.6	122	64	-47.5
3	-2.14	168	120	-28.6
3	-1.59	201	130	-35.3
3	-0.29	121	105	-13.2
3	-0.79	142	114	-19.7
4	-2.17	138	108	-21.7
3	-4.77	153	96	-37.3
3	-4.91	180	135	-25
4	3.86	166	117	-29.5
3	-1.62	165	134	-18.8
3	4.39	167	134	-19.8
-1	3.36	151	86	-43.1
3	-1.96	139	116	-16.6
2	-11	90	34	-62.2
3	-3.74	112	74	-33.9
3	-1.21	121	82	-32.2
2	-5.5	209	154	-26.3
4	3.88	160	108	-32.5
3	-1.31	178	119	-33.2
-1	2.87	149	111	-25.5
4	1.23	142	102	-28.2
4	1.24	119	89	-25.2
4	2.83	63	29	-54
4	0.64	178	127	-28.7
3	1.67	171	130	-24
..	..	..	..	..
2	-4.66	183	134	-26.8
2	-1.14	196	148	-24.5
..	..	134	..	..
3	..	..	146	..
5	..	..	47	..
4	0.81	138	87	-37
2	1.82	..	142	..

Table A.2 Health indicators used in calculations for chapter 2, mid-1980s (cont.)

Country	Female life expectancy 1965	Female life expectancy 1986	% change in female life exp. 1965–86	Male life expectancy 1965	Male life expectancy 1986	% change in male life exp. 1965–86
Indonesia	45	58	28.89	43	55	27.91
Yemen Arab Rep.	38	47	23.68	37	44	18.92
Philippines	57	65	14.04	54	62	14.81
Morocco	51	62	21.57	48	58	20.83
Bolivia	47	55	17.02	42	52	23.81
Zimbabwe	50	60	20	46	56	21.74
Nigeria	43	52	20.93	40	49	22.5
Dominican Rep.	57	68	19.3	54	64	18.52
Papua New Guinea	44	54	22.73	44	51	15.91
Côte d'Ivoire	44	54	22.73	40	51	27.5
Honduras	52	66	26.92	48	62	29.17
Egypt	50	63	26	48	59	22.92
Nicaragua	52	63	21.15	49	60	22.45
Thailand	58	66	13.79	54	62	14.81
El Salvador	56	66	17.86	53	57	7.55
Botswana	49	62	26.53	46	56	21.74
Jamaica	67	76	13.43	64	71	10.94
Cameroon	47	58	23.4	44	54	22.73
Guatemala	50	63	26	48	58	20.83
Congo	51	60	17.65	48	56	16.67
Paraguay	67	69	2.99	63	65	3.17
Peru	52	62	19.23	49	59	20.41
Turkey	55	67	21.82	52	62	19.23
Tunisia	52	65	25	51	61	19.61
Ecuador	57	68	19.3	55	64	16.36
Mauritius	63	70	11.11	59	63	6.78
Colombia	59	68	15.25	54	63	16.67
Chile	63	75	19.05	57	68	19.3
Costa Rica	66	76	15.15	63	71	12.7
Jordan	52	67	28.85	49	63	28.57
Syria	54	66	22.22	51	62	21.57
Lebanon	64	..	..	60	..	..
Brazil	59	68	15.25	55	62	12.73
Malaysia	60	71	18.33	56	67	19.64
South Africa	54	63	16.67	49	59	20.41
Mexico	61	72	18.03	58	65	12.07
Uruguay	72	74	2.78	65	68	4.62
Hungary	72	75	4.17	67	67	0
Poland	72	76	5.56	67	68	1.49
Portugal	69	76	10.14	63	70	11.11

Female minus male life expectancy 1986	*Female change minus male change in life expectancy*	*Infant mortality rate*		*% change in IMR 1965–86*
		1965	*1986*	
3	0.98	136	87	-36
3	4.77	200	152	-24
3	-0.78	72	46	-36.1
4	0.74	145	85	-41.4
3	-6.79	160	113	-29.4
4	-1.74	103	74	-28.2
3	-1.57	177	104	-41.2
4	0.78	110	67	-39.1
3	6.82	140	64	-54.3
3	-4.77	149	96	-35.6
4	-2.24	128	72	-43.8
4	3.08	172	88	-48.8
3	-1.3	121	65	-46.3
4	-1.02	88	41	-53.4
9	10.31	120	61	-49.2
6	4.79	112	69	-38.4
5	2.5	49	19	-61.2
4	0.68	143	96	-32.9
5	5.17	112	61	-45.5
4	0.98	118	75	-36.4
4	-0.19	73	43	-41.1
3	-1.18	130	90	-30.8
5	2.59	152	79	-48
4	5.39	145	74	-49
4	2.93	112	64	-42.9
7	4.33	67	35	-47.8
5	-1.41	96	47	-51
7	-0.25	107	20	-81.3
5	2.45	72	18	-75
4	0.27	115	46	-60
4	0.65	114	50	-56.1
..	..	56	..	..
6	2.53	104	65	-37.5
4	-1.31	55	27	-50.9
4	-3.74	124	74	-40.3
7	5.96	82	48	-41.5
6	-1.84	48	28	-41.7
8	4.17	39	19	-51.3
8	4.06	42	18	-57.1
6	-0.97	65	18	-72.3

Table A.2 Health indicators used in calculations for chapter 2, mid-1980s (cont.)

Country	Female life expectancy		% change in female life exp. 1965–86	Male life expectancy		% change in male life exp. 1965–86
	1965	1986		1965	1986	
Yugoslavia	68	74	8.82	64	68	6.25
Panama	65	74	13.85	62	70	12.9
Argentina	69	74	7.25	63	67	6.35
Korea, Rep.	58	73	25.86	55	66	20
Algeria	51	63	23.53	49	60	22.45
Venezuela	65	73	12.31	61	66	8.2
Gabon	44	54	22.73	41	50	21.95
Greece	72	79	9.72	69	74	7.25
Oman	44	56	27.27	42	53	26.19
Trinidad and Tobago	67	72	7.46	63	67	6.35
Israel	74	77	4.05	71	73	2.82
Hong Kong	71	79	11.27	64	73	14.06
Singapore	68	75	10.29	64	70	9.38
Iran	52	59	13.46	53	59	11.32
Iraq	53	65	22.64	51	62	21.57
Romania	70	73	4.29	66	68	3.03
Saudi Arabia	50	65	30	47	61	29.79
Kuwait	65	75	15.38	61	71	16.39
United Arab Emirates	59	71	20.34	56	67	19.64
Libya	51	63	23.53	48	61	27.08
Spain	74	79	6.76	68	73	7.35
Ireland	73	76	4.11	69	71	2.9
New Zealand	74	77	4.05	68	71	4.41
Italy	73	79	8.22	68	74	8.82
United Kingdom	74	78	5.41	68	72	5.88
Belgium	74	78	5.41	68	72	5.88
Austria	73	77	5.48	66	70	6.06
Netherlands	76	80	5.26	71	74	4.23
France	75	80	6.67	68	74	8.82
Australia	74	80	8.11	68	75	10.29
Germany, Fed. Rep.	73	78	6.85	67	72	7.46
Finland	73	79	8.22	66	72	9.09
Denmark	75	78	4	71	73	2.82
Japan	73	81	10.96	68	75	10.29
Sweden	76	80	5.26	72	74	2.78
Canada	75	80	6.67	69	73	5.8
Norway	76	80	5.26	71	74	4.23
United States	74	79	6.76	67	71	5.97
Switzerland	75	80	6.67	69	74	7.25

.. Not available.
Source: See table A.5.

Female minus male life expectancy 1986	Female change minus male change in life expectancy	Infant mortality rate		% change in IMR 1965–86
		1965	1986	
6	2.57	72	27	-62.5
4	0.94	56	24	-57.1
7	0.9	58	33	-43.1
7	5.86	63	25	-60.3
3	1.08	154	77	-50
7	4.11	65	37	-43.1
4	0.78	153	105	-31.4
5	2.48	34	12	-64.7
3	1.08	174	103	-40.8
5	1.11	42	21	-50
4	1.24	27	12	-55.6
6	-2.79	28	8	-71.4
5	0.92	26	9	-65.4
0	2.14	157	109	-30.6
3	1.07	119	71	-40.3
5	1.26	44	26	-40.9
4	0.21	148	64	-56.8
4	-1.01	43	19	-55.8
4	0.7	100	33	-67
2	-3.55	138	85	-38.4
6	-0.6	38	11	-71.1
5	1.21	25	9	-64
6	-0.36	20	11	-45
5	-0.6	36	10	-72.2
6	-0.48	20	9	-55
6	-0.48	24	10	-58.3
7	-0.58	28	10	-64.3
6	1.04	14	8	-42.9
6	-2.16	22	8	-63.6
5	-2.19	19	10	-47.4
6	-0.61	24	9	-62.5
7	-0.87	17	6	-64.7
5	1.18	19	8	-57.9
6	0.66	18	6	-66.7
6	2.49	13	6	-53.9
7	0.87	24	8	-66.7
6	1.04	17	9	-47.1
8	0.79	25	10	-60
6	-0.58	18	7	-61.1

Table A.3 Health indicators used in calculations for chapter 2, mid-1960s and mid-1980s

Country	*Child mortality rate* 1965	*Child mortality rate* 1986	*% change in child mortality rate 1965–86*	*Total fertility rate* 1965	*Total fertility rate* 1986
Ethiopia	132	121	-8.33	5.8	6.3
Bhutan	115	78	-32.17	6	5.7
Burkina Faso	168	111	-33.93	6.4	6.5
Nepal	115	78	-32.17	6	5.9
Bangladesh	103	78	-24.27	6.8	5.6
Malawi	186	132	-29.03	7.8	7.6
Zaire	110	69	-37.27	6	6.1
Mali	198	147	-25.76	6.5	6.5
Myanmar	57	24	-57.89	5.8	4.4
Mozambique	149	115	-22.82	6.8	6.1
Madagascar	65	33	-49.23	6.6	6.4
Uganda	90	74	-17.78	6.9	6.9
Burundi	113	87	-23.01	6.4	6.5
Tanzania	108	77	-28.7	6.6	7
Togo	113	64	-43.36	6.5	6.5
Niger	146	107	-26.71	6.8	7
Benin	131	82	-37.4	6.8	6.5
Somalia	132	121	-8.33	6.7	6.8
Central African Rep.	131	105	-19.85	4.5	5.7
India	110	55	-50	6.2	4.4
Rwanda	113	95	-15.93	7.5	8
China	36	12	-66.67	6.4	2.3
Kenya	80	44	-45	8	7.7
Zambia	87	51	-41.38	6.6	6.8
Sierra Leone	214	147	-31.31	6.4	6.5
Sudan	127	77	-39.37	6.7	6.6
Haiti	103	61	-40.78	6.2	4.8
Pakistan	110	63	-42.73	7.2	6.8
Lesotho	63	39	-38.1	5.8	5.8
Ghana	90	61	-32.22	6.8	6.3
Sri Lanka	27	10	-62.96	4.8	2.9
Mauritania	137	100	-27.01	6.5	6.5
Senegal	146	104	-28.77	6.4	6.5
Afghanistan	194	166	-14.43	7.1	6.7
Chad	149	105	-29.53	6	5.9
Guinea	60	119	98.33	5.9	6
Kampuchea	72	72	0	6.2	4.7
Lao PDR	86	56	-34.88	6.2	5.9
Viet Nam	74	26	-64.86	6.7	4.5
Liberia	138	95	-31.16	6.4	6.6
Yemen PDR	171	86	-49.71	7	6.6

% change in total fertility rate 1965–86	Maternal mortality rate early 1980s	Lifetime % chance of maternal mortality
8.62	2000	14.16
-5	..	..
1.56	..	..
-1.67	850	5.86
-17.65	600	3.96
-2.56	250	2.26
1.67	800	5.71
0	..	..
-24.14	135	0.71
-10.29	479	3.45
-3.03	300	2.28
0	300	2.46
1.56	..	..
6.06	370	3.07
0	476	3.65
2.94	581	4.78
-4.41	1680	12.38
1.49	1100	8.63
26.67	600	4.03
-29.03	500	2.61
6.67	210	2
-64.06	44	0.12
-3.75	510	4.61
3.03	140	1.14
1.56	450	3.46
-1.49	607	4.71
-22.58	367	2.1
-5.56	600	4.79
0	..	..
-7.35	1400	10.11
-39.58	90	0.31
0	119	0.92
1.56	530	4.06
-5.63	640	5.03
-1.67	..	..
1.69	..	..
-24.19	..	..
-4.84	..	..
-32.84	110	0.59
3.12	173	1.36
-5.71	100	0.79

Table A.3 Health indicators used in calculations for chapter 2, mid-1960s and mid-1980s (cont.)

Country	*Child mortality rate* 1965	*Child mortality rate* 1986	*% change in child mortality rate* 1965–86	*Total fertility rate* 1965	*Total fertility rate* 1986
Indonesia	93	46	-50.54	5.5	3.6
Yemen Arab Rep.	171	86	-49.71	6.8	6.8
Philippines	48	29	-39.58	6.8	4.6
Morocco	95	39	-58.95	7.1	4.5
Bolivia	121	69	-42.98	6.6	6.1
Zimbabwe	72	44	-38.89	8	6
Nigeria	142	76	-46.48	6.9	6.9
Dominican Rep.	59	19	-67.8	6.9	3.8
Papua New Guinea	72	23	-68.06	6.2	5.2
Côte d'Ivoire	114	53	-53.51	7.4	7.1
Honduras	82	40	-51.22	7.4	5.7
Egypt	133	42	-68.42	6.8	4.6
Nicaragua	66	34	-48.48	7.2	5.6
Thailand	38	10	-73.68	6.3	3
El Salvador	33	26	-21.21	6.7	4.9
Botswana	56	27	-51.79	6.9	6.6
Jamaica	18	5	-72.22	5.4	3
Cameroon	109	65	-40.37	5.2	6.9
Guatemala	96	43	-55.21	6.7	5.8
Congo	82	45	-45.12	5.7	6.4
Paraguay	41	20	-51.22	6.6	4.6
Peru	84	37	-55.95	6.7	4.1
Turkey	63	17	-73.02	5.8	3.7
Tunisia	84	29	-65.48	7	4.4
Ecuador	54	26	-51.85	6.8	4.5
Mauritius	27	6	-77.78	4.8	2.2
Colombia	49	23	-53.06	6.5	3.2
Chile	18	4	-77.78	4.8	2.5
Costa Rica	24	4	-83.33	6.3	3.3
Jordan	53	13	-75.47	7.2	6
Syria	59	15	-74.58	7.7	6.9
Lebanon	18	10	-44.44	6.2	3.4
Brazil	43	24	-44.19	5.6	3.5
Malaysia	24	9	-62.5	6.3	3.5
South Africa	..	..	..	6.1	4.5
Mexico	38	22	-42.11	6.7	3.7
Uruguay	6	3	-50	2.8	2.6
Hungary	1.3	0.5	-61.54	1.8	1.8
Poland	1.3	0.6	-53.85	2.5	2.3
Portugal	5.2	0.9	-82.69	3.1	1.7

% change in total fertility rate 1965–86	*Maternal mortality rate early 1980s*	*Lifetime % chance of maternal mortality*
-34.55	800	3.41
0	..	..
-32.35	80	0.44
-36.62	327	1.75
-7.58	480	3.46
-25	145	1.04
0	1500	11.76
-44.93	56	0.26
-16.13	1000	6.08
-4.05	..	..
-22.97	82	0.56
-32.35	500	2.73
-22.22	65	0.44
-52.38	270	0.97
-26.87	74	0.43
-4.35	250	1.96
-44.44	102	0.37
32.69	303	2.48
-13.43	105	0.73
12.28	..	..
-30.3	469	2.56
-38.81	314	1.54
-36.21	207	0.92
-37.14	1000	5.17
-33.82	220	1.18
-54.17	52	0.14
-50.77	126	0.48
-47.92	55	0.16
-47.62	26	0.1
-16.67	..	..
-10.39	280	2.29
-45.16	..	..
-37.5	154	0.65
-44.44	59	0.25
-26.23	550	2.93
-44.78	92	0.41
-7.14	56	0.17
0	28	0.06
-8	12	0.03
-45.16	15	0.03

Table A.3 Health indicators used in calculations for chapter 2, mid-1960s and mid-1980s (cont.)

Country	*Child mortality rate* 1965	1986	*% change in child mortality rate 1965–86*	*Total fertility rate* 1965	1986
Yugoslavia	3.5	0.9	-74.29	2.7	2
Panama	32	10	-68.75	5.7	3.2
Argentina	13	6	-53.85	3.1	3.2
Korea, Rep.	20	7	-65	4.8	2.2
Algeria	94	33	-64.89	7.4	6.1
Venezuela	26	8	-69.23	6.1	3.8
Gabon	120	74	-38.33	4.1	5.3
Greece	1.3	..	..	2.3	1.8
Oman	171	63	-63.16	7.2	6.9
Trinidad and Tobago	9	3	-66.67	4.3	2.9
Israel	1.1	0.5	-54.55	3.8	2.9
Hong Kong	9	2	-77.78	4.5	1.9
Singapore	8	2	-75	4.7	1.7
Iran	87	54	-37.93	7.8	5.6
Iraq	64	27	-57.81	7.2	6.7
Romania	2.1	..	..	1.9	2
Saudi Arabia	103	29	-71.84	7.3	7.1
Kuwait	19	3	-84.21	7.4	4.8
United Arab Emirates	38	7	-81.58	6.8	5.7
Libya	86	39	-54.65	7.4	6.9
Spain	..	..	..	2.9	1.8
Ireland	1.0	0.4	-60.00	4	2.5
New Zealand	..	0.6	..	3.6	1.9
Italy	1.4	0.5	-64.29	2.7	1.5
United Kingdom	0.9	0.4	-55.56	2.9	1.8
Belgium	1.0	0.6	-40.00	2.6	1.5
Austria	1.3	0.4	-69.23	2.7	1.5
Netherlands	1.0	..	..	3	1.5
France	0.9	0.5	-44.44	2.8	1.8
Australia	1.0	0.4	-60.00	3	1.9
Germany, Fed. Rep.	1.1	0.4	-63.64	2.5	1.3
Finland	0.9	0.3	-66.67	2.4	1.7
Denmark	0.9	0.5	-44.44	2.6	1.4
Japan	1.4	0.5	-64.29	2	1.8
Sweden	0.6	0.3	-50.00	2.4	1.7
Canada	1.0	0.5	-50.00	3.1	1.7
Norway	0.9	0.5	-44.44	2.9	1.6
United States	0.9	0.6	-33.33	2.9	1.9
Switzerland	..	0.4	..	2.6	1.5

.. Not available.
Source: See table A.5.

% change in total fertility rate 1965–86	*Maternal mortality rate early 1980s*	*Lifetime % chance of maternal mortality*
-25.93	27	0.06
-43.86	90	0.35
3.23	85	0.33
-54.17	34	0.09
-17.57	129	0.94
-37.7	65	0.3
29.27	124	0.79
-21.74	12	0.03
-4.17	..	..
-32.56	..	..
-23.68	5	0.02
-57.78	6	0.01
-63.83	11	0.02
-28.21	..	..
-6.94	..	..
5.26	175	0.42
-2.74	52	0.44
-35.14	13	0.07
-16.18	..	..
-6.76	..	..
-37.93	11	0.02
-37.5	7	0.02
-47.22	14	0.03
-44.44	13	0.02
-37.93	..	..
-42.31	10	0.02
-44.44	11	0.02
-50	5	0.01
-35.71	13	0.03
-36.67	11	0.03
-48	11	0.02
-29.17	5	0.01
-46.15	4	0.01
-10	15	0.03
-29.17	4	0.01
-45.16	2	0
-44.83	4	0.01
-34.48	9	0.02
-42.31	5	0.01

Table A.4 Health inputs used in calculations for chapter 2, mid-1960s and mid-1980s

Country	Population per physician 1965	Population per physician 1984	Change in population per physician 1965–84	Population per nurse 1965	Population per nurse 1984	Change in population per nurse 1965–84
Ethiopia	70190	77360	10.22	5970	5290	-11.39
Bhutan	..	23310	..	..	2990	..
Burkina Faso	73960	57180	-22.69	4150	1680	-59.52
Nepal	46180	32710	-29.17	87650	4680	-94.66
Bangladesh	8100	6730	-16.91	..	8980	..
Malawi	47320	11560	-75.57	..	3130	..
Zaire	35130	13430	-61.77	..	1740	..
Mali	51510	25390	-50.71	3360	1350	-59.82
Myanmar	11860	3740	-68.47	11370	900	-92.08
Mozambique	18000	37950	110.83	5370	5760	7.26
Madagascar	10620	10000	-5.84	3650	1730	-52.6
Uganda	11110	21900	97.12	3130	2060	-34.19
Burundi	55910	21120	-62.23	7320	3040	-58.47
Tanzania	21700	..	..	2100	..	..
Togo	23240	8720	-62.48	4990	1240	-75.15
Niger	65540	38770	-40.85	6210	450	-92.75
Benin	32390	15940	-50.79	2540	1750	-31.1
Somalia	36840	16090	-56.32	3950	1530	-61.27
Central African Rep.	34020	23070	-32.19	3000	2170	-27.67
India	4880	2520	-48.36	6500	1700	-73.85
Rwanda	72480	34680	-52.15	7450	3650	-51.01
China	1600	1000	-37.5	3050	1700	-44.26
Kenya	13280	10100	-23.95	1930	950	-50.78
Zambia	11380	7100	-37.61	5820	740	-87.29
Sierra Leone	16840	13630	-19.06	4470	1090	-75.62
Sudan	23500	10110	-56.98	3360	1250	-62.8
Haiti	14000	7180	-48.71	12890	2290	-82.23
Pakistan	..	2900	..	9910	4900	-50.55
Lesotho	20060	18610	-7.23	4700	..	..
Ghana	13740	14890	8.37	3730	640	-82.84
Sri Lanka	5820	5520	-5.15	3220	1290	-59.94
Mauritania	36470	12110	-66.79	..	1200	..
Senegal	21130	13450	-36.35	2640	2090	-20.83
Afghanistan	15770	..	..	24430	..	..
Chad	72480	38360	-47.08	13610	3390	-75.09
Guinea	54430	57390	5.44	4750	6380	34.32
Kampuchea	22410	..	..	3670	..	..
Lao PDR	26510	4200	-84.16	5320	..	..
Viet Nam	..	1000	..	..	620	..
Liberia	12360	9240	-25.24	2290	1360	-40.61
Yemen PDR	12870	4340	-66.28	1850	1060	-42.7

% births with trained health worker 1984	% one-year-olds with DPT immunization		Change in % one-year-olds with DPT immunization 1981–86
	1981	1986	
58	6	16	166.67
3	13	27	107.69
..	2	34	1600
10	16	46	187.5
..	1	9	800
59	66	55	-16.67
..	18	36	100
27	..	8	..
97	5	23	360
28	56	51	-8.93
62	40	30	-25
..	9	39	333.33
12	38	73	92.11
74	58	81	39.66
15	9	41	355.56
47	6	5	-16.67
34	..	52	..
2	2	25	1150
..	12	24	100
33	31	58	87.1
..	17	78	358.82
..	..	75	..
..	..	75	..
..	44	66	50
..	44	66	50
25	15	30	100
20	1	29	2800
20	14	20	42.86
24	3	62	1966.7
28	56	77	37.5
73	22	37	68.18
87	45	61	35.56
23	18	32	77.78
..	..	53	..
..	3	25	733.33
..	..	12	..
..	..	15	..
47	..	37	..
..	7	28	300
99	..	51	..
89	39	28	-28.21

Table A.4 Health inputs used in calculations for chapter 2, mid-1960s and mid-1980s (cont.)

Country	*Population per physician* 1965	*Population per physician* 1984	*Change in population per physician 1965–84*	*Population per nurse* 1965	*Population per nurse* 1984	*Change in population per nurse 1965–84*
Indonesia	31700	9460	-70.16	9490	1260	-86.72
Yemen Arab Rep.	58240	6270	-89.23	..	2680	..
Philippines	..	6700	..	1130	2740	142.5
Morocco	12120	15610	28.8	2290	920	-59.83
Bolivia	3300	1540	-53.33	3990	2480	-37.84
Zimbabwe	8010	6700	-16.35	990	1000	1.01
Nigeria	29530	7980	-72.98	6160	1020	-83.44
Dominican Rep.	1700	1760	3.53	1640	1210	-26.22
Papua New Guinea	12640	6160	-51.27	620	890	43.55
Côte d'Ivoire	20640	..	..	2000	..	..
Honduras	5370	1510	-71.88	1530	670	-56.21
Egypt	2300	790	-65.65	2030	800	-60.59
Nicaragua	2560	1500	-41.41	1390	530	-61.87
Thailand	7160	6290	-12.15	4970	710	-85.71
El Salvador	..	2830	..	1300	930	-28.46
Botswana	27460	6910	-74.84	17720	700	-96.05
Jamaica	1990	2060	3.52	340	490	44.12
Cameroon	26720	13990	-47.64	5830	1950	-66.55
Guatemala	3690	2180	-40.92	8250	850	-89.7
Congo	14210	8140	-42.72	950	570	-40
Paraguay	1850	1460	-21.08	1550	1000	-35.48
Peru	1650	1040	-36.97	900	1010	12.22
Turkey	2900	1380	-52.41	2290	1030	-55.02
Tunisia	8000	2150	-73.12	1150	370	-67.83
Ecuador	3000	830	-72.33	2320	620	-73.28
Mauritius	3930	1900	-51.65	2030	580	-71.43
Colombia	2500	1190	-52.4	890	630	-29.21
Chile	2100	1230	-41.43	600	370	-38.33
Costa Rica	2010	960	-52.24	630	450	-28.57
Jordan	4710	1140	-75.8	1810	1300	-28.18
Syria	5400	1260	-76.67	..	1440	..
Lebanon	1010	510	-49.5	2030	..	..
Brazil	2500	1080	-56.8	3100	1210	-60.97
Malaysia	6220	1930	-68.97	1320	1010	-23.48
South Africa	2050	..	..	490	..	..
Mexico	2080	1240	-40.38	980	880	-10.2
Uruguay	880	510	-42.05	590	190	-67.8
Hungary	630	310	-50.79	240	170	-29.17
Poland	800	490	-38.75	410	190	-53.66
Portugal	1240	410	-66.94	1160	..	..

% births with trained health worker 1984	*% one-year-olds with DPT immunization*		*Change in % one-year-olds with DPT immunization 1981–86*
	1981	*1986*	
31	..	69	..
12	25	14	-44
..	51	73	43.14
..	43	78	81.4
36	13	24	84.62
69	39	77	97.44
..	24	20	-16.67
57	27	80	196.3
34	50	41	-18
20	42	71	69.05
50	38	58	52.63
24	82	82	0
..	23	43	86.96
33	52	80	53.85
35	42	53	26.19
52	64	86	34.38
89	39	81	107.69
..	5	45	800
19	42	16	-61.9
..	42	71	69.05
22	28	58	107.14
44	18	42	133.33
78	64	71	10.94
60	36	89	147.22
27	26	51	96.15
84	82	85	3.66
51	20	58	190
95	97	93	-4.12
93	83	91	9.64
75	81	89	9.88
37	14	70	400
45	..	91	..
73	47	57	21.28
82	54	59	9.26
..	..	..	..
..	41	62	51.22
..	57	70	22.81
99	99	99	0
..	95	97	2.11
..	75	96	28

Table A.4 Health inputs used in calculations for chapter 2, mid-1960s and mid-1980s (cont.)

Country	Population per physician 1965	Population per physician 1984	Change in population per physician 1965–84	Population per nurse 1965	Population per nurse 1984	Change in population per nurse 1965–84
Yugoslavia	1200	550	-54.17	850	260	-69.41
Panama	2130	980	-53.99	1600	390	-75.62
Argentina	600	370	-38.33	610	980	60.66
Korea, Rep.	2700	1170	-56.67	2990	590	-80.27
Algeria	8590	2330	-72.88	11770	330	-97.2
Venezuela	1210	700	-42.15	560	..	..
Gabon	..	2790	..	760	270	-64.47
Greece	710	350	-50.7	600	450	-25
Oman	23790	1700	-92.85	6420	770	-88.01
Trinidad and Tobago	3810	960	-74.8	560	260	-53.57
Israel	400	350	-12.5	300	110	-63.33
Hong Kong	2520	1070	-57.54	1220	240	-80.33
Singapore	1900	1310	-31.05	600	340	-43.33
Iran	3800	2690	-29.21	4170	1050	-74.82
Iraq	5000	1740	-65.2	2910	1660	-42.96
Romania	760	570	-25	400	280	-30
Saudi Arabia	9400	690	-92.66	6060	320	-94.72
Kuwait	790	640	-18.99	270	200	-25.93
United Arab Emirates	..	1010	..	..	390	..
Libya	3850	690	-82.08	850	350	-58.82
Spain	800	320	-60	1220	260	-78.69
Ireland	950	680	-28.42	170	140	-17.65
New Zealand	820	580	-29.27	570	80	-85.96
Italy	1850	230	-87.57	790	250	-68.35
United Kingdom	870	680	-21.84	200	120	-40
Belgium	700	330	-52.86	590	110	-81.36
Austria	720	390	-45.83	350	180	-48.57
Netherlands	860	450	-47.67	270	170	-37.04
France	830	320	-61.45	380	110	-71.05
Australia	720	440	-38.89	150	110	-26.67
Germany, Fed. Rep.	640	380	-40.63	500	230	-54
Finland	1300	440	-66.15	180	60	-66.67
Denmark	740	400	-45.95	190	60	-68.42
Japan	970	660	-31.96	410	180	-56.1
Sweden	910	390	-57.14	310	100	-67.74
Canada	770	510	-33.77	190	120	-36.84
Norway	790	450	-43.04	340	60	-82.35
United States	670	470	-29.85	310	70	-77.42
Switzerland	710	700	-1.41	270	130	-51.85

.. Not available.
Source: See table A.5.

% births with trained health worker 1984	*% one-year-olds with DPT immunization*		*Change in % one-year-olds with DPT immunization 1981–86*
	1981	*1986*	
..	90	90	0
83	49	73	48.98
..	46	75	63.04
65	61	76	24.59
..	33	66	100
82	54	54	0
92	..	48	..
..	95	82	-13.68
60	9	77	755.56
90	52	79	51.92
99	84	92	9.52
99	84	94	11.9
100	87	98	12.64
82	29	74	155.17
60	13	76	484.62
99	..	90	..
78	53	89	67.92
99	54	94	74.07
96	45	75	66.67
76	55	62	12.73
96	..	88	..
..	36	45	25
99	72	72	0
..	..	88	..
98	44	67	52.27
100	95	95	0
..	90	90	0
..	97	95	-2.06
..	79	97	22.78
99	..	..	..
..	80	93	16.25
..	92	94	2.17
..	85	89	4.71
100	..	83	..
100	99	99	0
99	..	..	..
100	..	85	..
100	..	24	..
..	..	90	..

Table A.5 Notes and definitions for tables A.1 through A.4

Variable	*Source*	*Units*
Region	Created	
Country	WDR88[a]	
Population	WDR88, Ross and others 1988	Millions
GNP per capita	WDR88	U.S. dollars
GNP	Calculated	Millions of U.S. dollars
GDP	WDR88	Millions of U.S. dollars
Consumption, percent	WDR88	Percent
Government consumption, percent	WDR88	Percent
Medical care consumption	WDR88	Percent
Central government health, percentage of budget	WDR88	Percent
Government expenditure as percentage of GNP	WDR88	Percent
Total health spending per capita	Calculated	U.S. dollars
Central government spending on health per capita	Calculated	U.S. dollars
Approximate private medical spending per capita	Calculated	U.S. dollars
Female life expectancy at birth, 1965	WDR88	Years
Female life expectancy at birth, 1986	WDR88	Years
Percentage change in female life expectancy at birth, 1965–86	Calculated	Percent

Explanation

Asia = 1; Africa = 2; Europe, Middle East, North Africa = 3; Latin America and the Caribbean = 4; Industrial = 5: Classification of countries for summary tables in chapter 2.

Name of the country; sorted in same order as in WDR88.

Population, 1986, table 1; missing values filled in from Ross and others 1988.

GNP per capita, 1986, table 1.

Total GNP 1986 (population times per capita GNP).

GDP 1986, table 2.

Private consumption as percentage of GDP, 1986, table 5.

Government consumption as percentage of GDP, 1986, table 5. If in private consumption, this entry is 0.

Government and private consumption devoted to medical care (ICP), 1980–85, table 6. ICP = International Comparison Project. These numbers are derived from purchasing power parity consumption estimates. For details see Kravis and others 1982.

Central government expenditure on health, 1986, table 23. For many countries this number does not capture substantial expenditures for health at other levels of government.

Total central government expenditure as percentage of GNP, 1986, table 23.

Approximated using ICP medical consumption percentage applied to GDP per capita.

Calculated from government spending and GNP figures cited above.

Very imprecise. Total spending less central government spending per capita. Some values are negative.

Female life expectancy at birth, 1965, table 33.

Female life expectancy at birth, 1986, table 33.

Calculated from the previous two entries.

Table A.5 Notes and definitions for tables A.1 through A.4 (cont.)

Variable	*Source*	*Units*
Male life expectancy at birth, 1965	WDR88	Years
Male life expectancy at birth, 1986	WDR88	Years
Percentage change in male life expectancy at birth, 1965–86	Calculated	Percent
Female minus male life expectancy at birth, 1986	Calculated	Years
Female change minus male change in life expectancy at birth, 1965–86	Calculated	Percent
Infant mortality rate, 1965	WDR88	Per 1,000 live births
Infant mortality rate, 1986	WDR88	Per 1,000 live births
Percentage change in infant mortality rate, 1965–86	Calculated	Percent
Child mortality rate, 1965	Ross and others 1988	Per 1,000 surviving one-year-olds
Child mortality rate, 1986[b]	Ross and others 1988	Per 1,000 surviving one-year-olds
Percentage change in child mortality rate, 1965–86	Calculated	Percent
Total fertility rate, 1965	WDR88	Number of children per woman
Total fertility rate, 1986	WDR88	Number of children per woman
Percentage change in total fertility rate, 1965–86	Calculated	Percent
Maternal mortality rate	WDR88, SWC88[c]	Per 100,000 live births
Lifetime chance of maternal mortality	Calculated	Percent

Explanation
Male life expectancy at birth, 1965, table 33.
Male life expectancy at birth, 1986, table 33.
Calculated from the previous two entries.
Excess of female life expectancy over male life expectancy. Negative numbers are atypical but do occur.
Excess improvement in female life expectancy relative to male life expectancy during 1965–86. Sensitive to changes in sex-specific IMR.
Infant mortality rate, 1965, table 33.
Infant mortality rate, 1986, table 33.
Calculated from the previous two entries.
Child death rate, 1965–70, table 32.
Child death rate, 1985–90, table 32.
Calculated from the previous two entries.
Total fertility rate, 1965, table 28.
Total fertility rate, 1986, table 28.
Calculated from the previous two entries.
Maternal mortality rate around 1980. Very imprecise. Includes pregnancy and delivery-related deaths, including abortion-related.
Combines chance of dying per birth (maternal mortality rate) and the expected number of children (total fertility) to estimate a woman's chance of dying in childbirth over her lifetime. Early 1980s.

Table A.5 Notes and definitions for tables A.1 through A.4 (cont.)

Variable	*Source*	*Units*
Population per physician, 1965	WDR88	Number of people
Population per physician, 1984	WDR88	Number of people
Change in population per physician, 1965–86	Calculated	Percent
Population per nursing person, 1965	WDR88	Number of people
Population per nursing person, 1984	WDR88	Number of people
Change in population per nursing person, 1965–86	Calculated	Percent
Births attended by trained health worker, 1984	WDR88	Percent
DPT immunization, 1981	SWC88	Percent
DPT immunization, 1986	SWC88	Percent
Percentage change in DPT immunization, 1981–86	Calculated	Percent

a. WDR88 = World Bank 1988c.

b. The child mortality rates for industrial countries are reported for 1985–87, with the exact year varying by country. The data for industrial countries for this period and for 1965 are from United Nations, Department of Economic and Social Affairs 1975 and 1991.

c. SWC88 = UNICEF 1988.

Explanation

Population per physician around 1965, table 29. Imprecise; definition varies across countries.

Population per physician around 1984, table 28. If value is missing for 1984, value for 1981 is used.

Calculated from the previous two entries.

Population per nurse, health worker, and trained midwife around 1965, table 29. Imprecise; definition varies across countries.

Population per nurse, health worker, and trained midwife around 1984, table 28. If value is missing for 1984, value for 1981 is used.

Calculated from the previous two entries.

Very imprecise. Births attended by trained health worker—including trained midwives but not traditional attendants—1984.

Very imprecise. Proportion of one-year-olds fully immunized against DPT in 1981.

Very imprecise. Proportion of one-year-olds fully immunized against DPT in 1986.

Calculated from the previous two entries.

Table A.6 GNP of selected Asian countries, 1975, 1980, 1985, and most recent year

(national currency units)

Country	Currency units	1975	1980	1985	Most recent year
Bangladesh	millions	125688	198208	425580	557846 (1987)
Bhutan	millions	..	1804	2315	2624 (1986)
China	millions	300600	433600	830600	1099000 (1987)
India	billions	742	1477	2426	3026 (1987)
Indonesia	billions	13004	46903	90560	92239 (1986)
Korea	billions	10065	36672	72850	99790 (1987)
Malaysia	millions	22625	51390	71838	69757 (1987)
Myanmar	millions	23470	38447	55499	56371 (1986)
Nepal	millions	17671	27894	524668	59673 (1987)
Papua New Guinea	millions	1004	1708	2292	2819 (1987)
Philippines	millions	134200	264500	594500	706300 (1987)
Sri Lanka	millions	26364	66095	161694	178724 (1986)
Thailand	millions	303300	653100	996800	1199200 (1987)

.. Not available.

Source: World Bank data.

Table A.7 Percentage of GNP devoted to government spending in selected Asian countries, 1975, 1980, 1985, and most recent year

Country	1975	1980	1985	Most recent year
Bangladesh	9.4	15.4	14.4	16.8
Bhutan	..	33.8	52.6	45.1
China	16.4	18.3	20.2	18.6
India	18.7	18.5	22.2	23.6
Indonesia	21.0	30.0	50.0	23.7
Korea	17.1	20.9	20.4	28.6
Malaysia	31.2	41.0	37.9	39.4
Myanmar	12.2	13.3	16.7	16.6
Nepal	11.4	14.6	18.7	19.3
Papua New Guinea	30.6	36.5	40.2	34.1
Philippines	13.4	15.7	15.5	19.1
Sri Lanka	24.3	35.8	33.4	30.0
Thailand	18.9	17.7	18.1	18.7

.. Not available.

Source: Tan and Mingat forthcoming, table B3.6. To maintain comparability with health expenditure data cited in other sources, minor changes or additions were made for China (World Bank data), Indonesia, and Papua New Guinea (JSI 1990). For Indonesia, the numbers for 1980 and 1985 are incorrect, but they are the only figures consistent with reported spending on health.

Table A.8 Government health spending in selected Asian countries, 1975, 1980, 1985, and most recent year
(millions of national currency units)

	Government health spending				*Government health spending as a percentage of GNP*			
Country	*1975*	*1980*	*1985*	*Most recent year*	*1975*	*1980*	*1985*	*Most recent year*
Bangladesh	573	1527	2429	3686	0.5	0.8	0.6	0.7
Bhutan	..	11	31	32	..	0.6	1.3	1.2
China	2170	3686	7387	8490	0.7	0.9	0.9	0.8
India	12000	17000	35000	48000	1.6	1.2	1.5	1.6
Indonesia	25000	340000	621000	832000	0.2	0.7	0.7	0.9
Korea	37000	200000	456000	619000	0.4	0.5	0.6	0.6
Malaysia	599	1115	1732	1870	2.6	2.2	2.4	2.7
Myanmar	195	329	595	638	0.8	0.9	1.1	1.1
Nepal	127	163	406	492	0.7	0.6	0.1	0.8
Papua New Guinea	27	55	81	97	2.6	3.2	3.5	3.4
Philippines	809	1373	3779	4512	0.6	0.5	0.6	0.6
Sri Lanka	410	1003	2031	2400	1.6	1.5	1.3	1.3
Thailand	1618	6129	12582	13700	0.5	0.9	1.3	1.1

.. Not available.

Source: Health spending—Bangladesh: BIDS 1988, World Bank data, Griffin 1989; Bhutan: World Bank 1989a; Myanmar: World Bank data; Burma, Department of Health 1987; China: World Bank data; India: Indian Institute of Management 1987, World Bank 1989b; Indonesia: World Bank data; Korea: World Bank data; Nepal: World Bank 1989c; Philippines: World Bank data; Sri Lanka: World Bank data; Thailand: World Bank data. These are the primary sources. Also see notes after table A.15 for details. Health spending as a percentage of GNP is calculated from tables A.6, A.7, and health spending in A.8.

Table A.9 Health spending by source in selected Asian countries, most recent year

(millions of national currency units)

	Government		Total				Spending as a percentage of GNP					
Country	Central	Other	Government	Private	Insurance	Total	Central govt.	Other govt.	Total govt.	Private	Insurance	Total
Bangladesh	3686	0	3686	5529	0	9215	0.7	0	0.7	1.0	0	1.7
Bhutan	32	0	32	19	0	51	1.2	0	1.2	0.7	0	2.0
China	362	8128	8490	13584	21816	43890	0.0	0.7	0.8	1.2	2.0	4.0
India	10000	38000	48000	77000	5000	129000	0.3	1.2	1.6	2.5	0.2	4.3
Indonesia	690000	142000	832000	1324000	68000	2224000	0.7	0.2	0.9	1.4	0.1	2.4
Korea	250000	369000	619000	3389000	1130000	5138000	0.3	0.4	0.6	3.4	1.1	5.1
Malaysia	1769	101	1870	561	2	2433	2.5	0.1	2.7	0.8	0	3.5
Myanmar	638	0	638	1148	0	1786	1.1	0	1.1	2.0	0	3.2
Nepal	492	0	492	320	0	811	0.8	0	0.8	0.5	0	1.4
Papua New Guinea	42	55	97	10	1	107	1.5	1.9	3.4	0.3	0	3.8
Philippines	3860	652	4512	11731	677	16920	0.5	0.1	0.6	1.7	0.1	2.4
Sri Lanka	2160	240	2400	1680	60	4140	1.2	0.1	1.3	0.9	0	2.3
Thailand	13700	0	13700	31236	274	45210	1.1	0	1.1	2.6	0	3.8

Source: Generally the same as table A.8, supplemented by data reported in background papers for Asian Development Bank 1987. For some categories in some countries the author has made estimates. See notes after table A.15 for details. Most recent year in GNP is calculated from table A.6.

Table A.10 Percentage of government budgets devoted to health in selected Asian countries, 1975, 1980, 1985, and most recent year

Country	*1975*	*1980*	*1985*	*Most recent year*
Bangladesh	5.0	5.0	4.0	3.9
Bhutan	..	1.8	2.5	2.7
China	4.4	4.6	4.4	4.2
India	8.7	6.3	6.6	6.7
Indonesia	0.9	2.4	1.4	3.8
Korea	2.1	2.6	3.1	2.2
Malaysia	8.5	5.3	6.4	6.8
Myanmar	6.8	6.4	6.4	6.8
Nepal	6.3	4.0	0.4	4.3
Papua New Guinea	8.7	8.8	8.8	10.0
Philippines	3.2	3.3	4.1	3.3
Sri Lanka	6.4	4.2	3.8	4.5
Thailand	2.8	5.3	7.0	6.1

.. Not available.
Source: Calculated from previous tables.

Table A.11 Exchange rates and population for selected Asian countries, 1975, 1980, 1985, and most recent year

	Exchange rates of national currencies against U.S. dollar				*Population (millions)*			
Country	*1975*	*1980*	*1985*	*Most recent year*	*1975*	*1980*	*1985*	*Most recent year*
Bangladesh	12.02	15.45	28.00	30.95	78.9	88.5	100.6	106.1
Bhutan	8.65	7.86	12.37	12.96	1.0	1.1	1.2	1.3
China	1.86	1.50	2.94	3.72	916.0	976.7	1040.3	1068.5
India	8.38	7.86	12.37	12.96	613.0	673.2	765.1	797.5
Indonesia	415.00	626.99	1110.58	1282.56	130.2	146.6	162.2	166.4
Korea	484.00	607.43	870.02	822.57	35.3	38.2	41.1	42.1
Malaysia	2.39	2.18	2.48	2.52	12.3	13.9	15.6	16.5
Myanmar	6.37	6.60	8.47	7.33	30.4	34.8	36.9	38.0
Nepal	11.00	12.00	18.25	21.82	12.8	14.6	16.5	17.6
Papua New Guinea	1.31	1.49	1.00	1.10	2.7	3.0	3.5	3.7
Philippines	7.25	7.51	18.61	20.57	43.1	49.0	54.7	58.4
Sri Lanka	7.01	16.53	27.16	28.02	13.5	14.7	15.8	16.1
Thailand	20.38	20.48	27.16	25.72	41.4	47.0	51.7	53.6

Source: Exchange rates: for Bhutan, World Bank 1989e; for all others, IMF 1987; population: World Bank, *World Development Report*, various years.

Table A.12 Health spending per capita for selected Asian countries, 1975, 1980, 1985, and most recent year
(U.S. dollars)

	Government spending			*Most recent year*					
				Government		*Total*			
Country	*1975*	*1980*	*1985*	*Central*	*Other*	*Govern-ment*	*Pri-vate*	*Insur-ance*	*Total*
Bangladesh	0.60	1.12	0.86	1.12	0.00	1.12	1.68	0.00	2.81
Bhutan	..	1.27	2.09	1.90	0.00	1.90	1.14	0.00	3.04
China	1.27	2.52	2.42	0.09	2.04	2.13	3.42	5.49	11.04
India	2.34	3.23	3.73	0.98	3.66	4.63	7.41	0.46	12.51
Indonesia	0.46	3.70	3.45	3.23	0.67	3.90	6.20	0.32	10.42
Korea	2.14	8.62	12.75	7.22	10.66	17.87	97.86	32.63	148.37
Malaysia	20.34	36.84	44.72	42.55	2.43	44.97	13.49	0.04	58.51
Myanmar	1.01	1.43	1.90	2.29	0.00	2.29	4.12	0.00	6.41
Nepal	0.90	0.93	1.35	1.28	0.00	1.28	0.83	0.00	2.11
Papua New Guinea	7.52	12.22	23.11	10.23	13.45	23.68	2.37	0.12	26.18
Philippines	2.59	3.73	3.71	3.21	0.54	3.76	9.77	0.56	14.09
Sri Lanka	4.33	4.13	4.73	4.79	0.53	5.32	3.72	0.13	9.18
Thailand	1.92	6.37	8.96	9.94	0.00	9.94	22.66	0.20	32.79

.. Not available.
Source: Calculated from previous tables.

Table A.13 Spending for health by source in selected Asian countries, most recent year
(percent)

	Government				
Country	*Central*	*Other*	*Total government*	*Private*	*Insurance*
Bangladesh	40.0	0.0	40.0	60.0	0.0
Bhutan	62.5	0.0	62.5	37.5	0.0
China	0.8	18.5	19.3	31.0	49.7
India	7.8	29.2	37.0	59.3	3.7
Indonesia	31.0	6.4	37.4	59.5	3.1
Korea	4.9	7.2	12.0	66.0	22.0
Malaysia	72.7	4.1	76.9	23.1	0.1
Myanmar	35.7	0.0	35.7	64.3	0.0
Nepal	60.6	0.0	60.6	39.4	0.0
Papua New Guinea	39.1	51.4	90.5	9.0	0.5
Philippines	22.8	3.9	26.7	69.3	4.0
Sri Lanka	52.2	5.8	58.0	40.6	1.4
Thailand	30.3	0.0	30.3	69.1	0.6

Source: Calculated from previous tables.

Table A.14 Allocation of government budget to inputs and services in selected Asian countries, most recent year
(percent; estimated)

Country	Most recent year	Inputs			Services	
		Salaries	Nonsalary	Capital	Hospitals	Clinics, primary, public health
Bangladesh	1987	51	23	26	56	44
China	1987	18	56	26	67	33
India	1983	51	42	7	71	29
Indonesia	1986	39	36	25	59	41
Korea	1986	8	57	35	50	50
Malaysia	1983	67	19	14	59	41
Myanmar	1986	29	36	35	33	67
Nepal	1987	53	37	10	50	50
Papua New Guinea	1986	68	28	4	43	57
Philippines	1985	43	51	6	58	42
Sri Lanka	1986	44	44	12	70	30
Thailand	1985	48	29	23	58	42

Source: See notes following table A.15.

Table A.15 Hospitals and hospital beds in selected Asian countries, most recent year

	Hospitals		*Hospital beds*		*Hospitals' average size*		*Total*	
Country	*Govern-ment*	*Private*	*Govern-ment*	*Private*	*Govern-ment*	*Private*	*Hospitals*	*Beds*
Bangladesh	397	0	25066	4500	63	n.a.	397	29566
China	66149	0	2296819	0	35	n.a.	66149	2296819
India	4093	3381	394553	141182	96	42	7474	535735
Indonesia	428	255	65741	29709	154	117	683	95450
Korea	143	370	13495	61893	94	167	513	75388
Malaysia	101	197	32495	5444	322	28	298	37939
Myanmar	620	0	25599	0	41	n.a.	620	25599
Nepal	80	11	3343	559	42	51	91	3902
Papua New Guinea	19	1	4778	15	251	15	20	4793
Philippines	612	1227	47861	42418	78	35	1839	90279
Sri Lanka	479	..	39759	4000	83	..	479	43759
Thailand	662	365	72342	8278	109	23	1027	80620

.. Not available.

n.a. Not applicable.

Source: See following notes.

Population per bed	*Beds owned by government (%)*	*Government health spending absorbed by hospitals (%)*	*Government spending* US$	*Government spending* As % of GNP	*Cost per bed (US$)*	*Per capita income (US$)*	*Multiple of per capita income per bed*	*Overall bed occ. rate*	*Cost per day occupied (US$)*	*Ratio of cost per day occupied to per capita income*
3589	85	56	1.12	0.66	2,661	160	17	67	10.88	0.068
465	100	67	2.13	0.77	665	300	2	91	2.00	0.007
1489	74	71	4.63	1.58	6,650	290	23	80	22.77	0.079
1743	69	59	3.90	0.90	5,822	490	12	55	29.00	0.059
558	18	50	17.87	0.62	27,881	2370	12	60	127.31	0.054
435	86	59	44.97	2.68	13,474	1830	7	63	58.59	0.032
1484	100	33	2.29	1.13	1,122	200	6	97	3.17	0.016
4511	86	50	1.28	0.82	3,371	150	22	70	13.19	0.088
772	100	43	23.68	3.42	7,886	720	11	68	31.77	0.044
647	53	58	3.76	0.64	2,658	560	5	77	9.46	0.017
368	91	70	5.32	1.34	1,508	400	4	84	4.92	0.012
665	90	58	9.94	1.14	4,270	810	5	80	14.62	0.018

Notes for tables A.6–A.15

Table A.7

Data for Bhutan for most recent year are for 1989 and are from World Bank 1991.

Tables A.8 and A.9

Bangladesh: BIDS 1988; health = 66% of total health and family welfare (calculated from Griffin 1989); private = 1.5, public = average for 5 years from ADB 1987.
Bhutan: Private assumed to be same proportion as in Nepal.
India: Private ratio from table 3.1 in Indian Institute of Management 1987; government for 1975 is from an internal World Bank report and is for 1976–77, and includes water and sanitation.
Indonesia: ADB 1987; 1975 and 1980 filled in from World Bank 1984 estimates and Ross and others 1988. Estimates of central government expenditure are higher in the former than in the latter.
Korea: Based on an internal World Bank report and Kwon 1987 projection.
Malysia: Ghazali and others 1987; updated using World Bank data and author's interpolations based on population and GNP growth rates.
Nepal: Private from Pannenborg 1988 and Daly 1987.
Philippines: Everything estimated based on ADB 1987, and Integrated Health Care Services 1987.
Papua New Guinea: JSI 1990; private, used lowest ratio in table (Malaysia).
Sri Lanka: Based on Jayasuriya 1987; Alailima and Mohideen 1984; and an internal World Bank report.
Thailand: Internal World Bank memorandum.
For Bangladesh, "Health in Government" 1975 is Central 1972 from World Bank 1984.
For Indonesia, "Health in Government" 1975, 1980 is Central 1972, 1981 from World Bank 1984.
For Philippines, "Health in Government" 1975 is Central 1972 from World Bank 1984.

Table A.14: Allocation to inputs

Bangladesh: Griffin 1989, calculated from table 6.
Myanmar: ADB 1987 country paper.
China: Estimated from World Bank data; Jamison and others 1984, table 3.7, p. 74.
India: Calculated from Rao, Kahn, and Prasad 1987, p. 33, weighted percentage from medical and public health only.
Indonesia: Calculated from World Bank data.
Korea: Calculated from ADB 1987; refers only to central subsidies to government health facilities; fairly meaningless.
Malaysia: Estimates from ADB 1987 background paper, and Westinghouse Health Systems and Government of Malaysia 1985. Latter gives central capital as 14%; other ratios based on ADB numbers for 1983.
Nepal: Daly 1987, table 4.
Papua New Guinea: Thomason and Newbrander 1988, figure 3 and appendix 1.
Philippines: ADB 1987.
Sri Lanka: World Bank data.
Thailand: Wibulpolprasert, Buapradubkul, and Chantrasatid 1987, p. 24; percentages assume the three categories exhaust expenditures.

Table A.14: Allocation to services

Bangladesh: Calculated from Griffin 1989, neglecting administration and education.
Myanmar: ADB 1987, appendix 3, assuming all allocated to tertiary, secondary, or primary.
China: World Bank data.
India: Calculated from Rao, Kahn, and Prasad 1987, table 3.4.
Indonesia: Calculated from World Bank data.
Korea: This is a guess. Information in Republic of Korea, Ministry of Health and Social Affairs 1986 indicates no hospital spending, but I assume medical aid and cities are in that category.
Malaysia: ADB 1987, appendix IV.
Nepal: Estimates by Pannenborg 1988, p. 22.
Papua New Guinea: Calculated from Thomason and Newbrander 1988, appendix 1, see services.
Philippines: Republic of the Philippines, Department of Health 1987, table 1, for 1985.
Sri Lanka: Quoted in ADB 1987 and internal World Bank report.

Table A.15: Hospitals and beds

Asian Development Bank 1987 and background papers for that publication, except data for Nepal, which are from Pannenborg 1988.

Table A.15: Government hospital occupancy rates

Bangladesh: Griffin 1989.
Myanmar: Barnum and Kutzin 1990.
China: Barnum and Kutzin 1990.
India: Indian Institute of Management 1987.
Indonesia: Barnum and Kutzin 1990.
Korea: Barnum and Kutzin 1990.
Malaysia: Martins 1989.
Nepal: Pure guess.
Papua New Guinea: JSI 1990.
Philippines: Integrated Health Care Services 1987.
Sri Lanka: World Bank data.
Thailand: Estimate, based on rural in Golladay 1980 = 64%.

Table A.16 Membership and national coverage of insurance plans in selected Asian countries, around 1985–86

Country and insurance plan	*Primary members (thousands)*	*Total coverage (thousands)*	*Population (thousands)*	*Labor force (thousands)*
Bangladesh	0	0	105868	29756
China				
GEIS	22530	22530		
Labor insurance				
State enterprise	105000	165000		
Town and village ent.	79400	123900		
Private	8000	12480		
Collective		310000		
Total medical	214930	633910	1069000	630000
India				
CGHS	850	3200		
ESIS	7300	28000		
NICL	40	40		
Rural				
Total medical	8190	31240	797000	299144
Indonesia				
ASKES	3300	13000		
ASTEK	2000	2000		
PKTK (or DUKM)	5	16		
Dana Sehat	0	50		
Total medical	3305	13066	169735	65007
Korea				
Industrial	4304	13289		
KMIC	1074	4329		
Occupational	271	1131		
Regional	608	608		
Medical aid	0	4386		
Total medical	6257	23743	42031	17164
Malaysia				
SOCSO	2600	2600		
EPF	4500	4500		
Private	45	250		
Total medical	45	250	16560	6351

Nonagricultural labor (percent)	Coverage of nonagricultural labor (percent)	Coverage of population (percent)
39	87.5	59.3
30	9.1	3.9
43	11.8	7.7
64	57.0	56.5
58	1.2	1.5

Table A.16 Membership and national coverage of insurance plans in selected Asian countries, around 1985–86 (cont.)

Country and insurance plan	*Primary members (thousands)*	*Total coverage (thousands)*	*Population (thousands)*	*Labor force (thousands)*
Myanmar	347	347	38410	17023
Nepal	0	0	17444	7041
Papua New Guinea				
Public service assoc.	10	10	3494	1721
Philippines				
GSIS	1200	4700		
SSS	3300	15600		
Private/firm				
Total medical	4500	20300	58279	20395
Sri Lanka				
NIC and ICSL	50	50		
Private	40	40		
Total medical	90	90	16362	6009
Thailand				
Workmen's comp.	1108	1108		
Private	2	8		
Rural	0	1600		
Government	450	1800		
Public enterprise	66	262		
Free care	0	10750		
Total medical	518	14420	53535	27232

Source: China: Blendon 1979, Prescott and Jamison 1984, Wen and Hays 1976, and World Bank data; India: Indian Institute of Management 1987, Indian Society of Health Administrators 1984, International Social Security Association 1982 and 1983a, Seth and Gupta 1987, and Wadhawan 1987; Indonesia: Helminiak and Andreano 1987, REACH 1986a, 1986b, and 1987, Wasisto and others 1987, and World Bank data; Korea: Chung and Chung 1988, Federation of Korean Medical Insurance Societies 1986, International Social Security Association 1983b, Kim and others 1986, Kim 1987, Lee 1984, Republic of Korea, Ministry of Health and Social Affairs 1986, and World Bank data; Malaysia: Ghazali, Salam, and Baba 1987; Nepal: Pande 1987; Philippines: ADB 1987, INTERCARE 1987, International Social Security Association 1982 and 1983b, Philippines 1987, and REACH 1988; Papua New Guinea: Thomason and others 1987; Sri Lanka: Jayasuriya 1987; and Thailand: Wibulpolprasert, Buapradubkul, and Chantrasatid 1987.

Nonagricultural labor (percent)	Coverage of nonagricultural labor (percent)	Coverage of population (percent)
47	4.3	0.9
7	0.0	0.0
24	2.4	0.3
48	46.0	34.8
47	3.2	0.6
29	6.6	26.9

Table A.17 Expenditures per member, contributions, and coverage of insurance plans in selected Asian countries, around 1985–86

Country and insurance plan	Expenditure per member (medical)	Contribution (percent of wage)	Benefits: Outpatient	Benefits: Inpatient	Benefits: Maternity	Benefits: Dependents
China						
GEIS	84 yuan	5	free	free	—	no coverage
Labor insurance						
State enterprise	80 yuan	—	free	free	—	copay
Town and village ent.	80 yuan	—	free	free	—	copay
Private	—	3+	—	—	—	—
Collective	—	—	copay	copay	—	copay
India						
CGHS	326 Rs.	—	—	—	—	—
ESIS	260 Rs.	5-7.25	free	free	—	free
NICL	—	—	—	—	—	—
Rural	—	—	—	—	—	—
Indonesia						
ASKES	—	2	free	free	free	free
ASTEK	—	—	industrial accidents only	—	—	—
PKTK (or DUKM)	—	<5	free	free	free	free
Dana Sehat	—	<1	free	none	none	free
Korea						
Industrial	—	3-8	copay	copay	copay	copay
KMIC	—	3-8	copay	—	copay	—
Regional	—	—	copay	—	—	—
Medical aid	0	—	copay	copay	copay	copay
Malaysia						
SOCSO	—	2.25	accidents	accidents	no	no coverage
EPF	—	20	no	no	no	no coverage
Private	—	varies	varies	varies	varies	varies
Myanmar	63 kyats	2-3	—	—	—	no coverage

Table A.17 Expenditures per member, contributions, and coverage of insurance plans in selected Asian countries, around 1985–86 (cont.)

Country and insurance plan	*Expenditure per member (medical)*	*Contribution (percent of wage)*	*Benefits*			
			Out-patient	*In-patient*	*Mater-nity*	*Depen-dents*
Papua New Guinea						
Public service assoc.	—	—	life and accident	—	—	—
Philippines						
GSIS	—	—	no	partial	no	no
SSS	—	—	no	partial	no	no
Private/firm	—	—	varies	varies	varies	varies
Sri Lanka						
NIC and ICSL	—	—	no	yes	no	no
Private	—	—	varies	varies	varies	varies

— Could not be determined from available sources.

Note: For dependents, "no coverage" indicates that they receive no benefits. Entries other than "no coverage" indicate the terms of their coverage.

Source: China: Blendon 1979, Prescott and Jamison 1984, Wen and Hays 1976, and World Bank data; India: Indian Institute of Management 1987, Indian Society of Health Administrators 1984, International Social Security Association 1982 and 1983a, Seth and Gupta 1987, and Wadhawan 1987; Indonesia: Helminiak and Andreano 1987, REACH 1986a, 1986b, and 1987, Wasisto and others 1987, and World Bank data; Korea: Chung and Chung 1988, Federation of Korean Medical Insurance Societies 1986, International Social Security Association 1983b, Kim and others 1986, Kim 1987, Lee 1984, Republic of Korea, Ministry of Health and Social Affairs 1986, and World Bank data; Malaysia: Ghazali, Salam, and Baba 1987; Nepal: Pande 1987; Philippines: ADB 1987, INTERCARE 1987, International Social Security Association 1982 and 1983b, Philippines 1987, and REACH 1988; Papua New Guinea: Thomason and others 1987; Sri Lanka: Jayasuriya 1987; and Thailand: Wibulpolprasert, Buapradubkul, and Chantrasatid 1987.

Table A.18 Inpatient spending in government hospitals, by condition, in Myanmar, most recent year

Disease category	*Cases (thousands)*	*Average stay (days)*	*Total patient days (thousands)*	*Total cost (thousands of U.S. dollars)*	*Cost per case (U.S. dollars)*	*Percent of spending on these conditions only*	*Percent of total spending on hospitals*
Malaria	110.8	6.3	697.9	2,211.6	20	23.4	7.7
Tuberculosis	14.5	25.7	373.1	1,182.5	81	12.5	4.1
Obstetrical							
Normal delivery	59.6	4.9	292.0	925.3	16	9.8	3.2
Abortion	28.1	4.3	120.9	383.0	14	4.1	1.3
Digestive							
Intestinal infections	49.9	4.5	224.6	711.7	14	7.5	2.5
Ulcer	14.9	9.2	137.0	434.1	29	4.6	1.5
Other	16.7	8.1	134.9	427.4	26	4.5	1.5
Fever	32.4	6.7	217.0	687.8	21	7.3	2.4
Accidents/injuries							
Trauma	18.2	6.9	125.9	398.9	22	4.2	1.4
Head injuries	10.7	6.1	65.1	206.5	19	2.2	0.7
Poisoning	13.0	4.7	61.1	193.7	15	2.0	0.7
Respiratory							
Pneumonia	19.2	5.6	107.6	341.1	18	3.6	1.2
Chronic bronchitis	15.3	8.4	128.6	407.7	27	4.3	1.4
Other	18.0	9.1	163.7	518.7	29	5.5	1.8
Skin infections	13.9	9.5	132.2	418.9		4.4	1.5
Subtotal	435.2		2,981.6	9,448.6		100.0	32.9
All other causes	328.8						

Note: Disease statistics are for 1981 and are from 435 out of 619 hospitals. Budgetary data are for the most recent year. Columns may not add to totals because of rounding.
Source: Burma, Department of Health 1987, using cost and expenditure calculations in this report (cost per patient day = $3.17).

Table A.19 Predicted overall health spending based on GNP per capita for selected Asian countries

			Per capita health expenditure (U.S. dollars)				Predicted per capita health expenditure as a fraction of actual spending		
Country	*Population (millions)*	*GNP per capita (U.S. dollars)*	*Actual*	*Predicted with full sample*	*Predicted without Korea or Malaysia*	*Predicted without Bangladesh or Nepal*	*Predicted with full sample*	*Predicted without Korea or Malaysia*	*Predicted without Bangladesh or Nepal*
Nepal	17.6	150	2.10	3.13	3.09	4.01	1.5	1.5	1.9
Bangladesh	106.1	160	2.81	3.40	3.37	4.33	1.2	1.2	1.5
Myanmar	38.0	200	6.40	4.55	4.53	5.61	0.7	0.7	0.9
India	797.5	290	12.50	7.40	7.43	8.66	0.6	0.6	0.7
China	1068.5	300	11.00	7.74	7.78	9.01	0.7	0.7	0.8
Sri Lanka	16.1	400	9.20	11.27	11.40	12.61	1.2	1.2	1.4
Indonesia	166.4	490	10.40	14.69	14.93	15.98	1.4	1.4	1.5
Philippines	58.4	560	14.10	17.49	17.84	18.67	1.2	1.3	1.3
Papua New Guinea	3.7	720	26.20	24.28	24.92	25.03	0.9	1.0	1.0
Thailand	53.6	810	32.80	28.32	29.15	28.72	0.9	0.9	0.9
Malaysia	16.5	1,830	58.50	82.17	86.20	74.37	1.4	1.5	1.3
Korea	42.1	2,370	148.40	115.19	121.59	100.56	0.8	0.8	0.7

Table A.19 Predicted overall health spending based on GNP per capita for selected Asian countries (cont.)

	Annual resources required to bring spending up to trend					
Country	*Predicted with full sample (millions of U.S. dollars)*	*Fraction of shortfall*	*Predicted without Korea or Malaysia (millions of U.S. dollars)*	*Fraction of shortfall*	*Predicted without Bangladesh or Nepal (millions of U.S. dollars)*	*Fraction of shortfall*
Nepal	18.1	0.01	17.5	0.01	33.7	0.02
Bangladesh	62.9	0.04	59.3	0.04	160.9	0.09
Myanmar	-70.1		-70.9		-29.9	
India	-4,066.6		-4,041.4		-3,061.6	
China	-3,487.6		-3,445.6		-2,125.6	
Sri Lanka	33.3	0.02	35.4	0.02	54.8	0.03
Indonesia	713.4	0.50	754.5	0.49	927.7	0.54
Philippines	197.8	0.14	218.3	0.14	266.9	0.16
Papua New Guinea	-7.1		-4.7		-4.3	
Thailand	-239.9		-195.8		-218.5	
Malaysia	390.5	0.28	457.0	0.30	261.8	0.15
Korea	-1,398.0		-1,128.8		-2,013.9	

Source: Calculated, see chapter 4.

Table A.20 Predicted government health spending based on GNP per capita for selected Asian countries

			Per capita government health expenditure (U.S. dollars)				*Predicted government per capita health expenditure as a fraction of actual spending*		
Country	*Population (millions)*	*GNP per capita (U.S. dollars)*	*Actual*	*Predicted with full sample*	*Predicted without Korea or China*	*Predicted without Bangladesh or Nepal*	*Predicted with full sample*	*Predicted without Korea or Malaysia*	*Predicted without Bangladesh or Nepal*
Nepal	17.6	150	1.28	1.47	1.26	1.80	1.15	0.98	1.41
Bangladesh	106.1	160	1.12	1.59	1.37	1.93	1.42	1.23	1.72
Myanmar	38	200	2.29	2.08	1.87	2.46	0.91	0.82	1.07
India	797.5	290	4.81	3.24	3.13	3.68	0.67	0.65	0.77
China	1068.5	300	4.24	3.38	3.28	3.82	0.80	0.77	0.90
Sri Lanka	16.1	400	5.40	4.77	4.89	5.23	0.88	0.91	0.97
Indonesia	166.4	490	4.02	6.08	6.48	6.51	1.51	1.61	1.62
Philippines	58.4	560	3.92	7.14	7.79	7.53	1.82	1.99	1.92
Papua New Guinea	3.7	720	23.79	9.65	11.04	9.90	0.41	0.46	0.42
Thailand	53.6	810	10.00	11.11	13.00	11.25	1.11	1.30	1.12
Malaysia	16.5	1,830	45.00	29.54	40.21	27.28	0.66	0.89	0.61
Korea	42.1	2,370	22.91	40.29	57.53	36.12	1.76	2.51	1.58

Table A.20 Predicted government health spending based on GNP per capita for selected Asian countries (cont.)

	Annual resources required to bring government spending up to trend					
Country	*Predicted with full sample (millions of U.S. dollars)*	*Fraction of shortfall*	*Predicted without Korea or Malaysia (millions of U.S. dollars)*	*Fraction of shortfall*	*Predicted without Bangladesh or Nepal (millions of U.S. dollars)*	*Fraction of shortfall*
Nepal	3.3	0.01	-0.4		9.1	0.01
Bangladesh	49.6	0.08	26.9	0.03	86.0	0.11
Myanmar	-8.2		-15.9		6.5	0.01
India	-1,251.6		-1,338.9		-897.7	
China	-924.2		-1,023.9		-446.0	
Sri Lanka	-10.2		-8.2		-2.8	
Indonesia	342.8	0.53	408.8	0.50	415.1	0.52
Philippines	187.9	0.29	226.2	0.28	211.0	0.27
Papua New Guinea	-52.3		-47.2		-51.4	
Thailand	59.6	0.09	160.6	0.20	66.9	0.08
Malaysia	-255.0		-79.1		-292.5	
Korea	731.7		1,457.5		556.3	

Source: Calculated, see chapter 4.

Figure A.1 Distribution of total spending on health and family welfare, India, 1983
(percent)

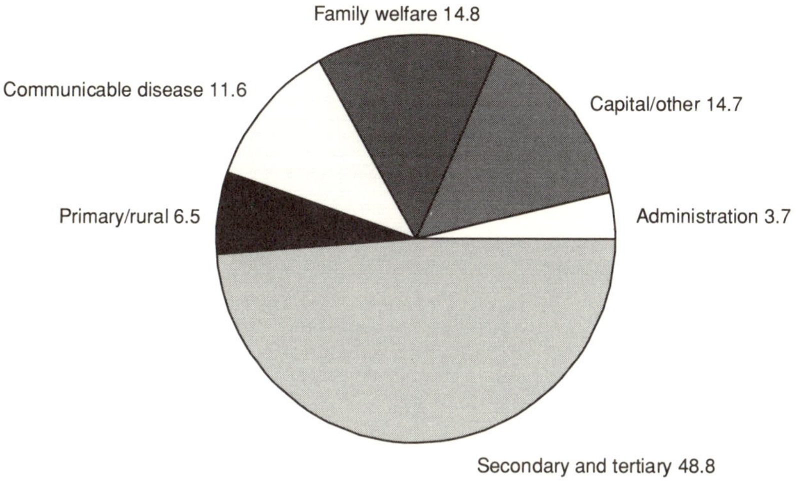

Source: Rao, Kahn, and Prasad 1987.

Figure A.2 Percentage of population living in rural areas and urban bias of total health and family welfare spending, by state, India, 1983

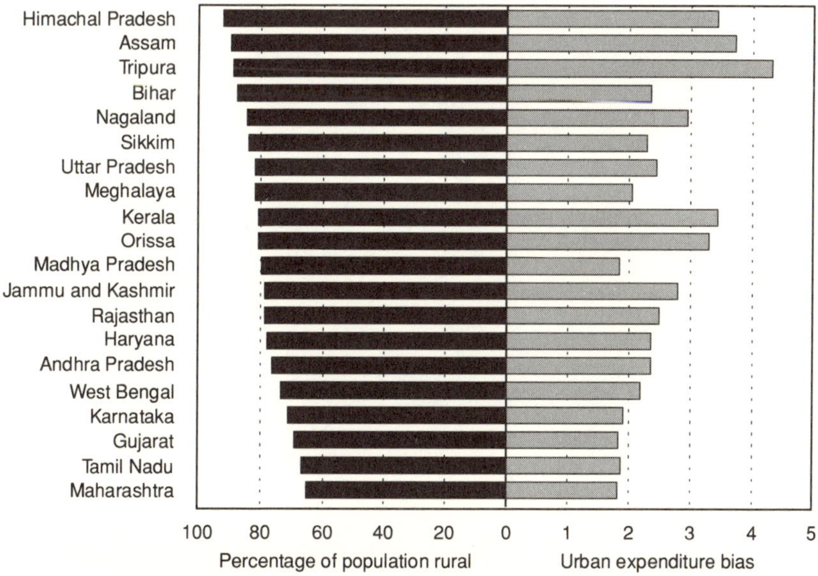

Source: Rao, Kahn, and Prasad 1987.

Figure A.3 Relation between provinces' income per capita and government health spending per capita, Indonesia, 1985
(thousands of rupiah)

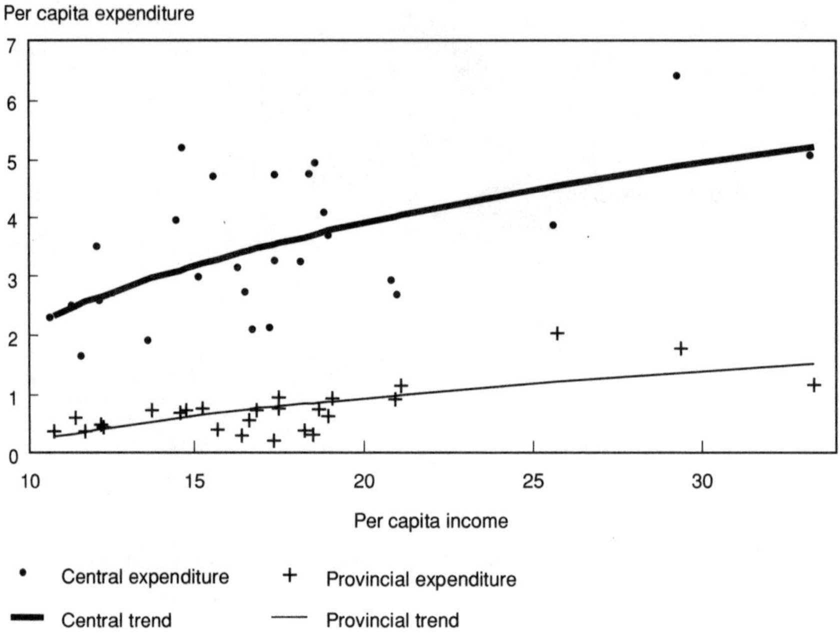

Source: World Bank data.

Figure A.4 Relation between provinces' infant mortality rates and government health spending per capita, Indonesia, 1985

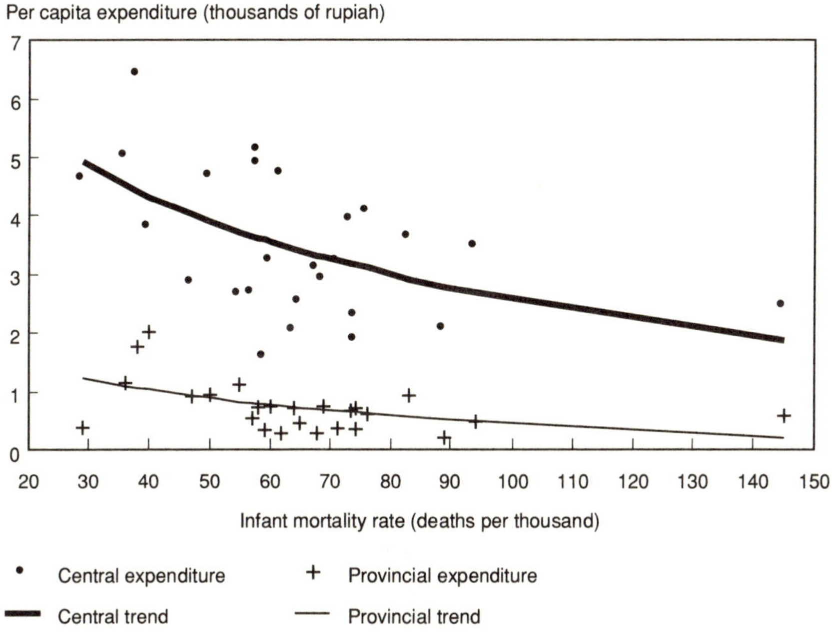

Source: World Bank data.

Figure A.5 Relation between provinces' health center paramedics per capita and income per capita, Indonesia, 1985

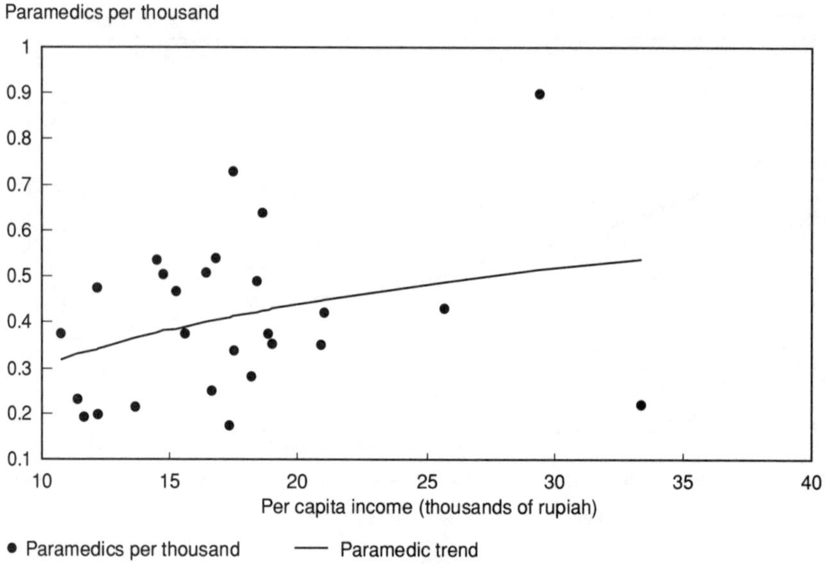

Source: World Bank data.

Figure A.6 Relation between provinces' health center paramedics per capita and infant mortality rates, Indonesia, 1985

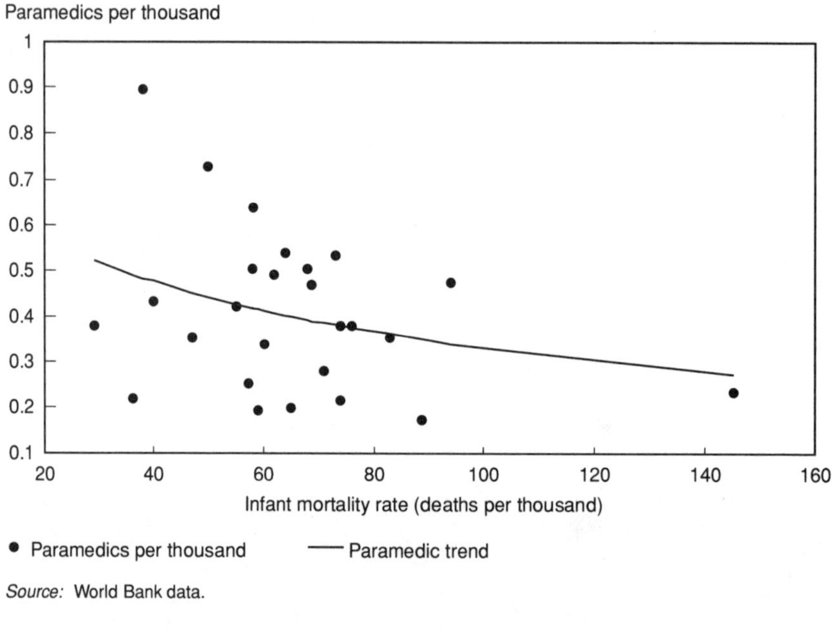

Source: World Bank data.

Figure A.7 Ministry of Health spending and per capita GNP by state, Malaysia, 1983
(Malaysian dollars)

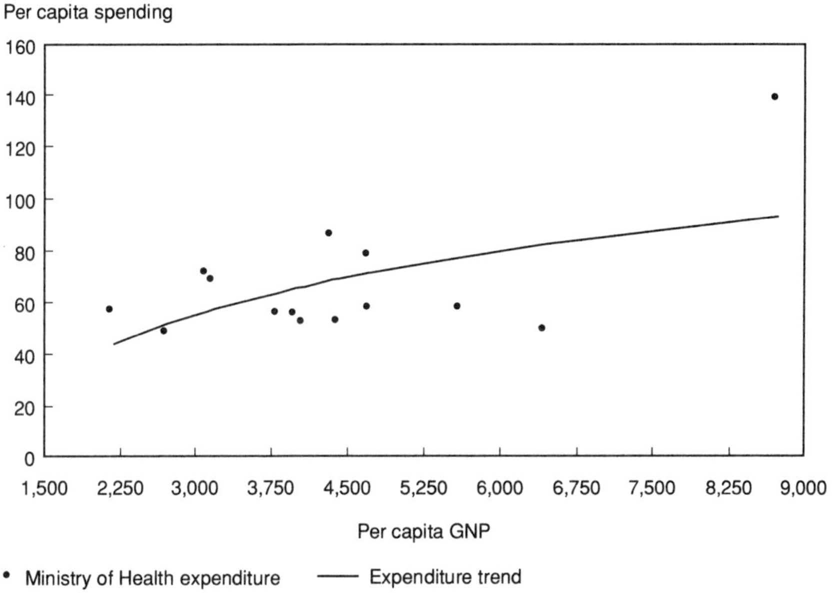

Source: Westinghouse Health Systems and Government of Malaysia 1985.

Figure A.8 Ministry of Health spending and infant mortality rates by state, Malaysia, 1983

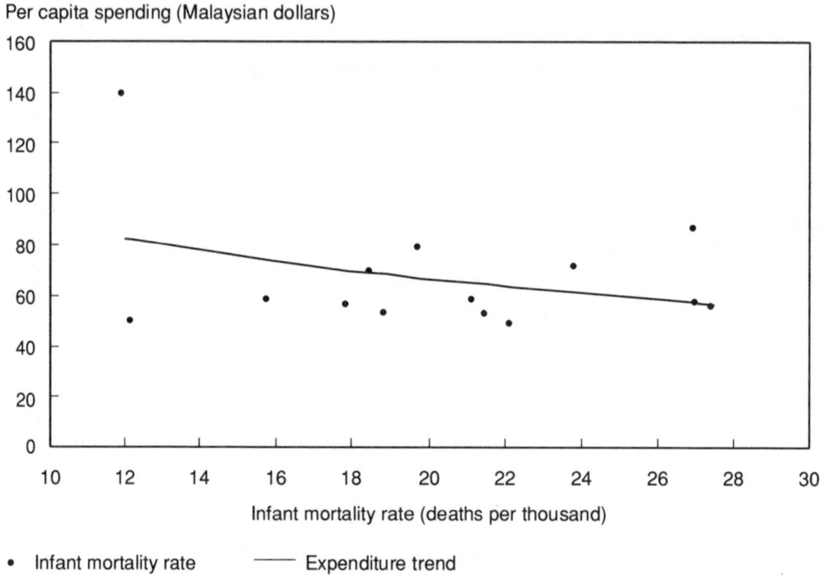

Source: Westinghouse Health Systems and Government of Malaysia 1985.

Figure A.9 Trends in total revenue budget and health spending, Bangladesh, 1978-88

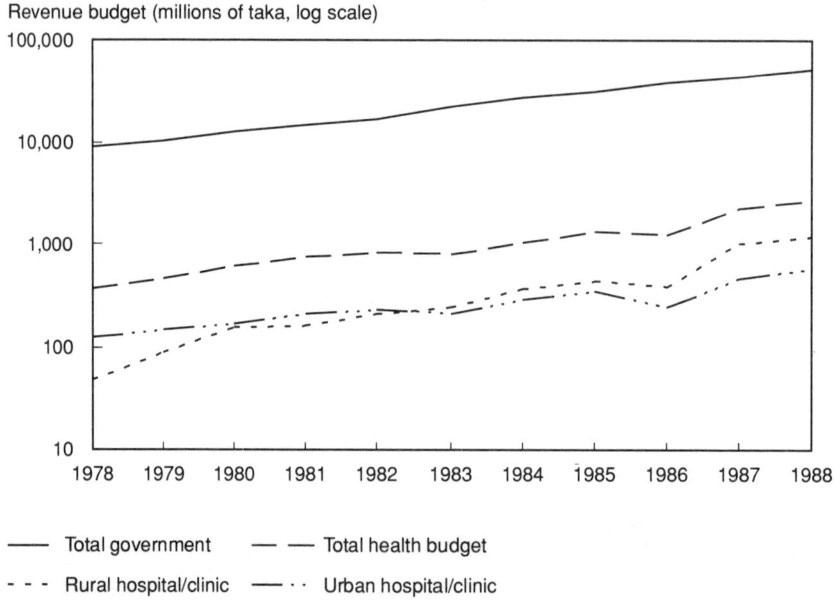

Source: IBA 1988.

Figure A.10 Percentage ill and percentage getting care, by age group, on day of 1987 household survey, rural Bangladesh, 1987

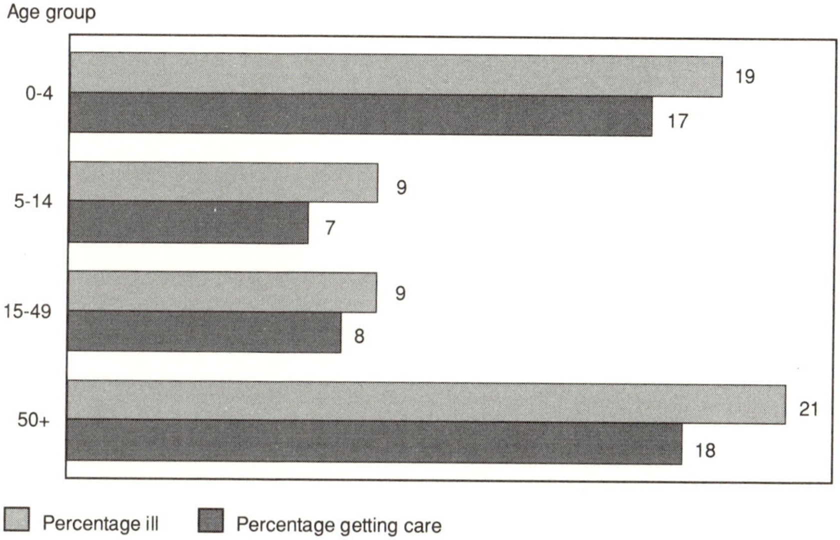

Source: BIDS 1988.

Figure A.11 Type of health care used by ill patients, by household landholdings, Bangladesh, 1987

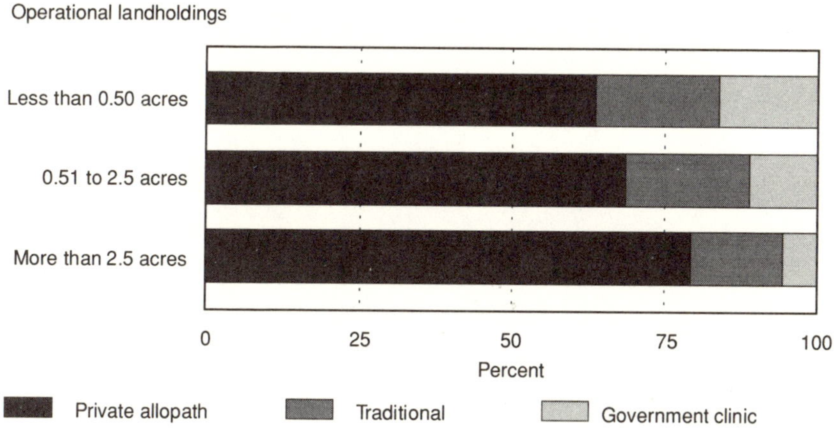

Source: BIDS 1988.

Bibliography

Abramson, Susan. 1986. "Willingness and Ability of the Poor to Pay for Health Care in Developing Countries." U.S. Agency for International Development, Washington, D.C. Draft.

Ahmad, Ehtisham, and Nicholas Stern. 1987. "Alternative Sources of Government Revenue: Illustrations from India, 1979–80." In David Newbery and Nicholas Stern, editors, *The Theory of Taxation for Developing Countries*. New York: Oxford University Press.

Ahmed, Ashraf U., and Mohammed A. Mabud. 1985. *Evaluation on Population Control Committee at Upazila Union and Ward Level*. Dhaka: University of Dhaka.

Ainsworth, Martha. 1984. "User Charges for Social Sector Finance: Policy and Practice in Developing Countries." CPD Discussion Paper 1984-6. World Bank, Washington, D.C.

Akin, John S. 1987. "Health Insurance in the Developing Countries: Prospects for Risk-Sharing." Paper prepared for the Asian Development Bank's Regional Seminar on Health Care Financing. World Bank, Washington, D.C.

Akin, John S., Charles C. Griffin, David K. Guilkey, and Barry M. Popkin. 1985. *The Demand for Primary Health Services in the Third World*. Totowa, N.J.: Rowman and Allanheld.

Alailima, P., and F. Mohideen. 1984. "Health Sector Expenditure Flows in Sri Lanka." *World Health Statistics Quarterly* 37:403–20.

Alfiler, Concepcion P. 1986. "Health Financing in the Philippines: A Review of the Literature." Paper prepared for the PIDS-UPSE workshop on Health Policy and Development, December 17–18. University of the Philippines College of Public Administration, Quezon City, Philippines.

Andreano, Ralph, and Thomas Helminiak. 1987. "The Role of the Private Sector in Health Care in the Developing Countries." Paper presented at the seminar on Health Care Financing, Asian Development Bank, Manila, Philippines, July 27–August 3.

Asian Development Bank. 1986. *Use of Rural Health Services*. Proceedings of the Regional Seminar on the Use of Rural Health Services, Manila, Philippines, January 20–25.

———. 1987. *Health Care Financing: Proceedings of the Regional Seminar on Health Care Financing 27 July – 3 August 1987*. Manila: Information Office, Asian Development Bank.

The bibliography contains many more sources than are cited in the text. It is intended as a listing of sources on health financing in Asia.

Bangladesh Institute of Development Studies (BIDS). 1988. *Bangladesh Health Finance and Expenditure Study*. Final report of a study conducted for the Director General of Health Services, Government of Bangladesh. Dhaka.

Barnum, Howard. 1985. "Nepal: Financial Tables for PHN Sector and Project Analysis." World Bank, Asia Region, Country Department I, Washington, D.C.

———. 1987. "Hospital Expenditure in Indonesia." World Bank, Population and Human Resources Department, Washington, D.C.

Barnum, Howard, and Joseph Kutzin. 1990. "Hospital Resource Use." World Bank, Population and Human Resources Department, Population, Health, and Nutrition Division, Washington, D.C.

Berman, Peter. 1985. *Equity and Cost in the Organization of Primary Health Care in Java, Indonesia*. Cornell International Agricultural Economics Study 23. Ithaca, N.Y.: Cornell University.

Berman, Peter A., Davidson R. Gwatkin, and Susan E. Burger. 1986. "Community-based Health Workers: Head Start or False Start Towards Health For All?" Department of Population, Health, and Nutrition Technical Note 86-3. World Bank, Washington, D.C.

Besley, T.J., D.L. Bevan, and P. Collier. 1985. "Why Might Health Insurance Contribute to a Cost Recovery Program?" Paper presented at the World Bank conference on Risk Sharing for Health Provision, Washington, D.C., December 17.

Birdsall, Nancy. 1986. "Cost Recovery in Health and Education: Bank Policy and Operations." Department of Population, Health, and Nutrition Technical Note 86-24. World Bank, Washington, D.C.

———. 1989. "Pragmatism, Robin Hood, and Other Themes: Good Government and Social Well-Being in Developing Countries." World Bank, Latin America and the Caribbean Regional Office, Country Department I, Washington, D.C.

Birdsall, Nancy, Francois Orivel, Martha Ainsworth, and Punam Chuhan. 1986. "Paying for Health and Schooling Services in Rural Africa: A Mali Case Study." Department of Population, Health, and Nutrition Technical Note 86-15. World Bank, Washington, D.C.

Blendon, J. Robert. 1979. "Can China's Health Care Be Transplanted without China's Economic Policies?" *New England Journal of Medicine* 300(26):1453–58.

Bulatao, Rodolfo A., Alan D. Lopez, and Patience Stevens. 1989. "World Estimates and Projections of Mortality by Cause, 1970–2015." World Bank, Population, and Human Resources Department, Population, Health, and Nutrition Division, Washington, D.C. Draft.

Burma, Department of Health. 1987. "Health Care Financing, Burma." Paper presented at the seminar on Health Care Financing, Asian Development Bank, Manila, the Philippines, July 27–August 3. Excerpted in Asian Development Bank (1987).

Burma, Ministry of Planning and Finance. 1982. *Five-Year Development Programme 1983/84 to 1987/88*. Volume I. Rangoon.

Chatterjee, Meera. 1990. *Indian Women: Their Health and Productivity*. World Bank Discussion Paper 109. Washington, D.C.

Chayovan, Napaporn, Peerasit Kamnuansilpa, and John Knodel. 1988. *Thailand Demographic and Health Survey 1987*. Bangkok: Institute of Population Studies, Chulalongkorn University, and Columbia, Md.: Institute for Resource Development, Westinghouse.

Chernichovsky, Dov, and Oey Astra Meesook. 1986. "Utilization of Health Services in Indonesia." *Social Science and Medicine* 23(6):611–20.

China, Department of Population Statistics of the State Statistical Bureau. 1986. *China In-Depth Fertility Survey, Phase I, Volume I*. Series CIDFS No. 4. Beijing.

China, Ministry of Public Health, Policy Research Office. 1986. *Studies on Several Policies Concerning the Reform of Health Work.* Beijing.

Chung, M.H., and K.K. Chung. 1988. "Successful Implementation of a Voluntary Community Health Insurance Programme in Korea." *Asia-Pacific Journal of Public Health* 2(1):63–71.

Cross, P.N., Maggie A. Huff, Jonathan D. Quick, and James A. Bates. 1986. "Revolving Drug Funds: Conducting Business in the Public Sector." *Social Science and Medicine* 22(3):335–43.

Daly, Patricia M. 1987. *Health Financing and Cost Recovery in Nepal.* Integrated Rural Health and Family Planning Services, Project No. 367-0135.

de Ferranti, David. 1983. "Health Sector Financing and Expenditure in Developing Countries: Current Issues." World Bank, Department of Population, Health and Nutrition, Washington, D.C.

———. 1984. "Strategies for Paying for Health Services in Developing Countries." Department of Population, Health, and Nutrition Technical Note GEN25. World Bank, Washington, D.C.

Dunlop, David W., B. Eilene Oldwine, Chung Kyong-Kyun, and Kim Bong-Young. 1982. *Korea Health Demonstration Project.* Project Impact Evaluation 36. Washington, D.C.: U.S. Agency for International Development.

Elkins, Henry, D. Nagabrahmam, S.C. Sharma, and George Varky. 1986. "Financial, Organization, and Managerial Problems of Community Health Projects in India." PRICOR, Chevy Chase, Md.

Federation of Korean Medical Insurance Societies. 1986. "Outline of Medical Insurance in Korea." Seoul.

Gertler, Paul, Luis Locay, and Warren Sanderson. 1986. "The Demand for Health Care in Peru: Lima and the Urban Sierra, 1984." Health Sector Analysis of Peru Technical Report. State University of New York at Stony Brook.

Ghazali, Azizan Aiyub, Haji Abduk Halim Bin Abdul Salam, and Akbar Bin Baba. 1987. "Health Care Financing: Malaysia." Paper prepared for the seminar on Health Care Financing, Asian Development Bank, Manila, Philippines, July 27–August 3.

Golladay, Frederick. 1980. *Health.* Sector Policy Paper. Washington, D.C.: World Bank.

Gray, R. 1974. "The Decline of Mortality in Ceylon and the Demographic Effects of Malaria Control." *Population Studies* (28):205–29.

Griffin, Charles C. 1987. "User Charges for Health Care in Principle and Practice." Department of Population, Health, and Nutrition Technical Note 87-16. World Bank, Washington, D.C.

———. 1989. "Mobilizing Resources for Health and Family Planning: 1987 Bangladesh Health Expenditure Study Summary Report." Bangladesh, Directorate of Health Services, Dhaka.

Griffin, Charles C., and Vicente Paqueo. 1985. "Description and Analysis of the Philippine Medical Care Plan." Carolina Population Center, Chapel Hill, N.C.

———. Forthcoming. "Distribution and Growth of the Public and Private Medical Sectors in the Philippines." In Kenneth Lee and Anne Mills, editors, *Health Economics Research in Developing Countries.* New York: Oxford University Press.

Hakulinen, T., H. Hansluwka, A.D. Lopez, and T. Nakada. 1986a. "Estimation of Global Mortality Patterns by Cause of Death." In Hansluwka and others (1986).

———. 1986b. "Global and Regional Mortality Patterns by Cause of Death in 1980." *International Journal of Epidemiology* 15(2):226–33.

Hansluwka, Harald. 1986a. "Mortality in South and East Asia: An Assessment of Achievement and Failure." In Hansluwka and others (1986).

———. 1986b. "The Epidemiological Situation in the ESCAP Region—Facts, Fallacies, and Implications." In United Nations (1986).

Hansluwka, H., A.D. Lopez, Y. Porapakkham, and P. Prasartkul, editors. 1986. *New Developments in the Analysis of Mortality and Causes of Death.* Bangkok: Amarin Press.

Heller, Peter S. 1982. "A Model of the Demand for Medical and Health Services in Peninsular Malaysia." *Social Science and Medicine* 16:267–84.

Helminiak, Thomas, and Ralph Andreano. 1987. "Financing Health Services: Some Speculation and an Example from Indonesia." Produced for the World Bank, Washington, D.C.

Hobcraft, J., J. McDonald, and S. Rutstein. 1985. "Demographic Determinants of Infant and Child Mortality: A Comparative Analysis." *Population Studies* 39(3).

Hsiao, William C. 1984. "Transformation of Health Care in China." *New England Journal of Medicine* 310 (14, April):932–36.

———. 1988. *The Incomplete Revolution: China's Health Care System Under Market Socialism.* Cambridge, Mass.: Harvard University School of Public Health.

Ignatius, Adi. 1988. "Beijing Boom. China's Birthrate Rises Again Despite a Policy of One-Child Families. Officials Adopt Harsher Penalties." *The Wall Street Journal*, 14 July.

Indian Institute of Management. 1987. *Study of Health Care Financing India.* Based on Case Studies in Maharashtra and West Bengal, Ahmedabad. Report for Asian Development Bank, Manila.

Indian Society of Health Administrators. 1984. *Financing of Health Services in India.* New Delhi.

Institute of Business Administration (IBA). 1988. *Bangladesh Health Finance and Expenditure Study.* Dhaka: University of Dhaka.

Institute for Resource Development, Westinghouse, and Sri Lanka, Janalekhanaha Sankhyalekhana Departamentuva. 1988. *Sri Lanka 1987: Demographic Health Survey: Summary Report.* Colombo: Department of Census and Statistics, Ministry of Plan Implementation.

Integrated Health Care Services, Inc. (Intercare). 1987. "Health Care Financing in the Philippines: A Country Study." For the Asian Development Bank, Manila.

International Labour Organization. 1987. "Health Insurance in Asia: Country Profiles." Paper presented at the seminar on Health Care Financing, Asian Development Bank, Manila, Philippines, July 27–August 3.

International Labour Organization, Social Security Department. 1987. *Health Insurance in Asia: Country Profiles.* Geneva.

International Monetary Fund. 1987. *International Financial Statistics Yearbook.* Washington, D.C.

International Social Security Association. 1982. *Medical Care under Social Security in Developing Countries.* Studies and Research 18. Geneva.

———. 1983a. *Improving Cost Effectiveness in Health Care.* Studies and Research 19. Geneva.

———. 1983b. *Report of the Round Table Meeting on the Extension of Medical Care Programmes Under Social Security.* New Delhi, India.

Jamison, Dean T. 1985. "China's Health Care System: Policies, Organization, Inputs, and Finance." In Scott B. Holstead, Julia A. Walsh, and Kenneth S. Warren, editors, *Good Health at Low Cost.* New York: Rockefeller Foundation.

Jamison, Dean T., John R. Evans, Timothy King, Ian Porter, Nicholas Prescott, and Andre

Prost. 1984. *China, The Health Sector.* Washington, D.C.: World Bank.

Jayasuriya, Rohan. 1987. "Health Care Financing in Sri Lanka." Paper presented at the seminar on Health Care Financing, Asian Development Bank, Manila, Philippines, July 27–August 3.

Jimenez, Emmanuel. 1987. *Pricing Policy in the Social Sectors: Cost Recovery for Education and Health in Developing Countries.* Baltimore, Md.: Johns Hopkins University Press.

John Snow, Inc. (JSI). 1990. *Papua New Guinea: Health Sector Financing Study Project Final Report Vols. I and II.* Prepared for the Papua New Guinea Department of Health. Boston, Mass.

Kawnine, A.B.M. Nazmul, and Humayun Shamsul Kabir. 1987. "Health Care Financing: Country Paper of Bangladesh." Paper presented at the seminar on Health Care Financing, Asian Development Bank, Manila, Philippines, July 27–August 3.

Kielmann, Arnfried A., and Carl E. Taylor. 1983. *Child and Maternal Health Services in Rural India: The Narangwal Experiment.* 2 volumes. Baltimore, Md.: Johns Hopkins University Press.

Kim, Il Soon, Seung Hum Yu, Han Joong Kim, Young Moon Chae, Kyung Yong Rhee, and Myong Sei Sohn. 1986. "Impact of Regional Health Insurance on Utilization of Medical Care by the Rural Population of Korea." *Yonsei Medical Journal* 27(2):138–46.

Kim, Young-Ju. 1987. "Health Care Financing in Korea." Paper presented at the seminar on Health Care Financing, Asian Development Bank, Manila, Philippines, July 27–August 3.

Korale, R.B.M. 1988. *Sri Lanka Demographic and Health Survey 1987.* Colombo: Department of Census and Statistics, Ministry of Plan Implementation, and Columbia, Md.: Institute for Resource Development, Westinghouse.

Korea Institute for Population and Health. 1986. *Introduction to Health Situation in Korea, with Special Reference to KIPH Health Research.* Seoul.

———. 1987. *Workshop on Health Resources and Management: Presentation and Discussion Materials.* Workshop at Saejong Hotel, Chunchon, Kangwon Province, August 27–28.

Kravis, Irving B., Alan Heston, and Robert Summers. 1982. *World Product and Income: International Comparisons of Real Gross Product.* Baltimore, Md.: Johns Hopkins University Press.

Krister, S.J. 1988. "India's Health." World Bank, India Country Department, Population, Human Resources, Urban, and Water Operations Division, Washington, D.C.

Kwon, Soonwon. 1987. "Trend in National Health Expenditure." Paper presented at workshop on Health Resources and Management, Korea Institute for Population and Health, Chunchon, Kangwon Province, Korea, August 27–28.

Lee, Kyu Sik. 1987. "Medical Security System." Paper presented at workshop on Health Resources and Management, Korea Institute for Population and Health, Chunchon, Kangwon Province, Korea, August 27–28.

Lee, Sung-Woo. 1984. "Introduction of Korean Health Plan: Organization and Financing." *World Hospitals* 20(3, August):26–30.

Liu, Xinming, and Guobo Huang. 1987. "Health Care Financing: China." Paper presented at the seminar on Health Care Financing, Asian Development Bank, Manila, Philippines, July 27–August 3.

Luthra, K.L. 1987. "Health Care Financing in Developing Countries: An Overview of the Issues." Paper presented at the seminar on Health Care Financing, Asian Development Bank, Manila, Philippines, July 27–August 3.

Mach, E.P., and B. Abel-Smith. 1983. *Planning the Finances of the Health Sector: A Manual for Developing Countries*. Geneva: World Health Organization.

Martins, Jose. 1989. "Malaysia Health Development and Efficient and Equitable Resource Allocation: Report by the World Bank." World Bank, Asia Technical Department, Population and Human Resources Division, Washington, D.C.

Martorell, Reynaldo, Joanne Leslie, and Peter Moock. 1984. "Characteristics and Determinants of Child Nutritional Status in Nepal." *American Journal of Clinical Nutrition* 39:74–86.

Measham, Anthony R. 1986. "Review of PHN Sector Work and Lending In Health, 1980–85." Department of Population, Health, and Nutrition Technical Note 86-14. World Bank, Washington, D.C.

Meerman, Jacob. 1979. *Public Expenditures in Malaysia: Who Benefits and Why*. New York: Oxford University Press.

Meesook, Oey A. 1984. *Financing and Equity in the Social Sectors in Indonesia. Some Policy Options*. World Bank Staff Working Paper 703. Washington, D.C.

Mitchell, Marc D., Jane A. Thomason, Dayl S. Donaldson, and Paul Garner. 1988. "The Cost of Rural Health Services in Papua New Guinea." New Guinea Department of Health, Boroko.

Moon, Ok-Ryun. 1987. "The National Health Insurance Policy in Korea." Paper prepared for the Eighth Formal Meeting of the Board Asia-Pacific Academic Consortium for Public Health. Seoul National University School of Public Health, Seoul, Korea.

Muller, Manon, and Mary Young. 1986. "Health Care in China: The Availability, Utilization, and Cost of County Hospitals." Department of Population, Health, and Nutrition Technical Note 86-16. World Bank, Washington, D.C.

Myers, Charles N., Dow Mongkolsmai, and Banyanne Causino. 1985. *Financing Health Services and Medical Care in Thailand*. Report prepared for the U.S. Agency for International Development, Bangkok, Thailand. Also Development Discussion Paper 209. Harvard Institute for International Development, Cambridge, Mass.

Newbery, David, and Nicholas Stern, editors. 1987. *The Theory of Taxation for Developing Countries*. New York: Oxford University Press.

Newbrander, William C. 1987. "Papua New Guinea's Expenditure on Hospitals: Policy and Practice since Independence." *Health Policy and Planning* 2(3):227–35.

Osteria, Trinidad S., and Ida M. Siason. 1985. "Alternative Strategies for Financing Primary Health Care: Lessons from Six Case Studies." Report prepared for the U.S. Agency for International Development Primary Health Care Operations Research Project (PRICOR). Center for Human Resources, Chevy Chase, Md.

Pande, B.R. 1987. "Health Care Financing Country Paper: Nepal." Paper presented at the seminar on Health Care Financing, Asian Development Bank, Manila, Philippines, July 27–August 3.

Pannenborg, Charles O. 1988. "Nepal: Social Sector Strategy Review, Health Family Planning and Nutrition Sector." World Bank, Asia Region, Country Department 1, Population and Human Resources Division, Washington, D.C.

Park, Chong Kee, and Ha Cheong Yeon. 1981. "Recent Developments in the Health Care System of Korea." *International Social Security Review* 2(28):151–67.

Parker, R.L. 1986. "Health Care Expenditures in a Rural Indian Community." *Social Science and Medicine* 22(1):23–27.

Phua, Kai Hong. 1987. "Saving for Health." *World Health Forum* 8:38–41.

Prescott, Nicholas, and Dean T. Jamison. 1984. "Health Sector Finance in China." *World Health Statistics Quarterly* 37(4):387–402.

———. 1985. "The Distribution and Impact of Health Resource Availability in China."

International Journal of Health Planning and Management 1(1):45–56.

Preston, S. 1980. "Causes and Consequences of Mortality Decline in Less Developed Countries During the 20th Century." In R. Easterlin, editor, *Population and Economic Change in Less Developed Countries*. New York: National Bureau of Economic Research.

Raffel, W. Marshall. 1984. Comparative Health Systems. Philadelphia, Penn.: Pennsylvania State University Press.

Rao, N. Bhaskara, M.E. Kahn, and C.V.S. Prasad. 1987. *Health Sector Expenditure Differentials in India*. Baroda, India: Operations Research Group for the Ministry of Health and Family Welfare.

Rashid, Saeed Ahmed, Inam Kazmi, S.H. Rizvi, and Shamsul Haq. 1987. "Health Care Financing in Pakistan." Paper presented at the seminar on Health Care Financing, Asian Development Bank, Manila, Philippines, July 27–August 3.

REACH. 1986a. "Health Care Financing in Indonesia." John Snow, Inc., Arlington, Va.

———. 1986b. "PERTAMINA: The Transition of Employee Health Benefits from State-Owned Industry to the Private Sector." John Snow, Inc., Arlington, Va.

———. 1987. "A Business Plan for Tugu Mandiri of Jakarta, Indonesia to Establish a Health Insurance and Health Maintenance Organization." John Snow, Inc., Arlington, Va.

———. 1988. "Trip Report Evaluation of Philippine Medicare System." John Snow, Inc., Arlington, Va.

Republic of Korea, Economic Planning Department. 1986. "Expansion of Medical Insurance During the 6th Plan Period." Seoul.

Republic of Korea, Ministry of Health and Social Affairs. 1986. *Major Policies and Programmes in Health and Social Welfare Services*. Seoul.

Republic of the Philippines, Department of Health. 1987. "Health Care Financing: Philippines." Paper presented at the seminar on Health Care Financing, Asian Development Bank, Manila, Philippines, July 27–August 3.

Republic of the Philippines, Social Security System. 1987. *Social Security Law 1986*. Quezon City, Metro Manila.

Robertson, Robert L. 1985. "Review of Literature on Costs of Health Services in Developing Countries." Department of Population, Health, and Nutrition Technical Note 85-21. World Bank, Washington, D.C.

Robertson, Robert L., Bernardo Barona, and Ricardo Pabon. 1977. "Hospital Cost Accounting and Analysis: The Case of Candelaria." *Journal of Community Health* (3):61–79.

Rosenthal, M. Marilynn. 1987. *Health Care in the People's Republic of China*. Boulder, Colo.: Westview Press.

Ross, John A., Marjorie Rich, Janet P. Molzan, and Michael Pensak. 1988. *Family Planning and Child Survival: 100 Developing Countries*. New York: Columbia University Center for Population and Family Health.

Rutstein, Shea Oscar. 1983. "Infant and Child Mortality: Levels, Trends and Demographic Differentials." WFS Comparative Studies 24. International Statistical Institute, Voorburg, Netherlands.

Schieber, George J. 1987. *Financing and Delivering Health Care: A Comparative Analysis of OECD Countries*. Paris: Organisation for Economic Co-operation and Development Publications Service.

Schwartz, J. Brad, John S. Akin, and Barry M. Popkin. 1988. "Price and Income Elasticities of Demand for Modern Health Care: The Case of Infant Delivery in the Philippines." *World Bank Economic Review* 2(1):49–76.

Seth, M., and O.P. Gupta. 1987. "Health Care Financing: India." Paper presented at the seminar on Health Care Financing, Asian Development Bank, Manila, Philippines, July 27–August 3.

Sharma, R.R. 1987. "Health Care Financing: Fiji." Paper presented at the seminar on Health Care Financing, Asian Development Bank, Manila, Philippines, July 27–August 3.

Shepard, Donald S., and Elisabeth R. Benjamin. 1986. "Mobilizing Resources for Health: The Role of User Fees in Developing Countries." Development Discussion Paper 234. Harvard Institute for International Development, Cambridge, Mass.

Stevens, Carl M. 1983. "Alternatives for Financing Health Services in Pakistan." U.S. Agency for International Development, Washington, D.C.

———. 1984. "Alternative Social-Financing Schemes for the Health Services in the Philippines, Regions V (Bicol) and VI (Western Visayas)." U.S. Agency for International Development, Washington, D.C.

Stinson, Wayne W. 1982. *Community Financing*. Washington, D.C.: American Public Health Association.

Stewart, Frances. 1987. "Monitoring and Statistics for Adjustment with a Human Face." In Giovanni A. Cornia, Richard Jolly, and Frances Stewart, editors, *Adjustment with a Human Face*. Oxford: Clarendon Press.

Stinson, Wayne W., Marty Pipp, La Rue Seims, and Pat Sayer. 1987. *Community Financing of Primary Health Care: The PRICOR Experience*. A Comparative Analysis. Chevy Chase, Md.: Center for Human Resources.

Stout, Susan A. 1989. "Changing Signals: Family Welfare Strategy in India." World Bank, India Country Department, Population, Human Resources, Urban, and Water Operations Division, Washington, D.C.

Tan, Jee-Peng, and Alain Mingat. Forthcoming. *Education in Asia: A Comparative Study of Cost and Financing*. Washington, D.C.: World Bank.

Tanskul, Orathip, Chanet Khumthong, Charles Nash Myers, and Chayada Siripirom. 1986. "Community Finance of Primary Health Care in Thailand." Report prepared for the U.S. Agency for International Development Primary Health Care Operations Research Project (PRICOR). Center for Human Resources, Chevy Chase, Md.

Thomason, J.A., D. Makavo, K.L. Loh, and R.L. Kolehmainen-Aitken. 1987. "Health Care Financing in Papua New Guinea." Paper presented at the seminar on Health Care Financing, Asian Development Bank, Manila, Philippines, July 27–August 3.

Thomason, Jane A., and William C. Newbrander. 1988. "A Survey of Papua New Guinea's Health Sector Financing and Expenditure." New Guinea Department of Health, Boroko.

Torrens, Paul R. 1986. *Current Status of Health Financing Programs in Indonesia*. Rosslyn, Va.: JSI.

U.S. Department of Health and Human Services, Social Security Administration. 1982. *Social Security Programs Throughout the World, 1981*. Washington, D.C.

———. 1986. *Social Security Programs Throughout the World, 1985*. Washington, D.C.

———. 1988. *Social Security Programs Throughout the World, 1987*. Washington, D.C.

United Nations. 1985. *Mortality and Health Issues: Overview of Country Studies and Implications for Health, Economic and Social Welfare Planning*. Asian Population Studies Series 71. Bangkok: Economic and Social Commission for Asia and the Pacific.

———. 1986. *Mortality and Health Issues in Asia and the Pacific*. Asian Population Studies Series 78. Bangkok: Economic and Social Commission for Asia and the Pacific.

United Nations Commission of the European Communities. 1987. *World Comparisons of Purchasing Power and Real Product for 1980: Phase IV of the International Comparison Project, Part Two: Detailed Results for 60 Countries*. New York: United Nations and Eurostat.

United Nations, Department of Economic and Social Affairs. 1975. *1974 Demographic Yearbook, 26th Edition*. New York.

———. 1991. *1989 Demographic Yearbook, 41st Edition*. New York.

United Nations International Children's Emergency Fund (UNICEF). 1986. *A Situation Analysis of Children and Women in Burma*. Rangoon, Burma.

———. 1988. *State of the World's Children 1988*. New York: Oxford University Press.

van de Walle, E., and J. Knodel. 1980. "Europe's Fertility Transition: New Evidence and Lessons for Today's Developing World." *Population Bulletin* (34).

Vogel, Ronald J. 1988. *Cost Recovery in the Health Care Sector: Selected Country Studies in West Africa*. World Bank Technical Paper 82. Washington, D.C.

Wadhawan, Sahdev K. 1987. "Health Insurance in India: The Case for Reform." *International Labour Review* 126(4, July–August):479–94.

Walsh, Julia. 1984. *India Health Sector Analysis*. Technologies for Primary Health Care (PRITECH) Project. Washington, D.C.: USAID.

———. 1988. *Establishing Health Priorities in the Developing World*. New York: United Nations Development Programme.

Wasisto, Broto, Ridwan Malik, Paramita Sudharto, and Oscar Gish. 1987. "Health Care Financing in Indonesia." Paper presented at the seminar on Health Care Financing, Asian Development Bank, Manila, Philippines, July 27–August 3.

Wen, Chi-Pang, and Charles W. Hays. 1976. "Health Care Financing in China." *Medical Care* 14(23, March):241–54.

Westinghouse Health Systems and the Government of Malaysia, Health Services Financing Study Task Force. 1985. *Malaysia Health Financing Study Final Report*. Manila, Philippines: Asian Development Bank.

Wibulpolprasert, Suwit, Panna Buapradubkul, and Ngamjit Chantrasatid. 1987. "Health Care Financing: Thailand." Paper presented at the seminar on Health Care Financing, Asian Development Bank, Manila, Philippines, July 27–August 3.

World Bank. 1983. *China: Socialist Economic Development. Volume 3. The Social Sectors: Population, Health, Nutrition, and Education*. Washington, D.C.

———. 1984. *World Development Report 1984*. New York: Oxford University Press.

———. 1986. *Financing Education in Developing Countries: An Exploration of Policy Options*. Washington, D.C.

———. 1987a. *Bangladesh: Promoting Higher Growth and Human Development*. A World Bank Country Study. Washington, D.C.

———. 1987b. *Financing Health Services in Developing Countries: An Agenda for Reform*. A World Bank Policy Study. Washington, D.C.

———. 1988a. *Education in Sub-Saharan Africa: Policies for Adjustment, Revitalization, and Expansion*. A World Bank Policy Study. Washington, D.C.

———. 1988b. *Papua New Guinea: Policies and Prospects for Sustained and Broad-Based Growth*. 2 volumes. Washington, D.C.

———. 1988c. *World Development Report 1988*. New York: Oxford University Press.

———. 1989a. *Bhutan: Development Planning in a Unique Environment*. Washington, D.C.

———. 1989b. *India: Recent Developments and Medium-Term Issues*. Washington, D.C.

———. 1989c. *Nepal: Policies for Improving Growth and Alleviating Poverty*. Washington, D.C.

———. 1989d. *World Development Report 1989*. New York: Oxford University Press.

———. 1989e. *World Tables, 1988–89 Edition*. Baltimore, Md.: Johns Hopkins University Press.

———. 1990. *Brazil: The New Challenge of Adult Health*. Washington, D.C.

———. 1991. *World Development Report 1991*. New York: Oxford University Press.

World Health Organization. 1987. *Economic Support for National Health for All Strategies*. Background document for the Fortieth World Health Assembly. Geneva: World Health Organization.

———. 1988. *World Health Statistics*. Geneva.

World Health Organization Regional Office for South-East Asia. 1985. *The Pyongyang Conference. Primary Health Care in Action*. SEARO Regional Health Papers 6. New Delhi.

———. 1987. *Development of Strategies and Approaches to Malaria Control in South-East Asia*. SEARO Technical Publications 9. New Delhi.

Wulf, Luc De. 1986. *International Experience in Budgetary Trends during Economic Development and Its Relevance for China*. World Bank Staff Working Paper 760. Washington, D.C.

Yeon, Ha Cheong. 1981. *Primary Health Care in Korea. An Approach to Evaluation*. Seoul: Korea Development Institute.

Yeon, Ha Cheong. 1985. "Who Gains and Who Loses: An Overview of Equity and Efficiency in Korea's Health Insurance System." Takemi Program in International Health, Harvard School of Public Health, Cambridge, Mass.

Zachariah, Kunniparampil C., and My T. Vu. 1988. *World Population Projections 1987–88 Edition: Short- and Long-Term Estimates*. Baltimore, Md.: Johns Hopkins University Press.